As a pastor's wife, it's always frustrated me that health and wellness is often considered women's territory. As if all that is good, healthy, and natural is for women; and what is bad, unhealthy and synthetic is for men. While Mom serves fresh veggies and organic chicken, Dad winks at the kids and sings of burgers and fries. Seriously – what message does that send our children? Men, especially Christian men, should be leading their families in all that's good for them, and that includes physical health and wellness…and essential oils!

Ron Corica, in his new book, *You Can Lead a Man to Oils,* has created a literal lifeboat for guys, and for the women who love them. He gives men "permission" to get on board by proving health isn't a "girl thing." And he teaches wives how they may be unwittingly perpetuating the falsehood.

With practical tips for creating a "couples culture" for essential oil events (like drop the girly invitations and verbiage), he helps women know how to make the oily world welcoming to men. And, personally, I love doing life, including my Young Living business, in partnership with my best friend – my husband!

While *You Can Lead a Man to Oils* seems to be written as a fun "tips for wives" type book, men, too, will find themselves laughing and nodding in agreement, as Ron uses real life examples and humor to touch on every argument they've likely already experienced! A must-read for every oily family!

Stacy McDonald
Young Living Crown Diamond

In my opinion, Ron Corica's book *You Can Lead a Man to Oils* is very informative, yet light enough to educate and keep the reader engaged. The topic covered is a much needed one in today's essential oil world, and it was a pleasure to read!

Verick Burchfield
Young Living Crown Diamond

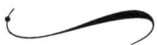

"Ron gives clear, easy to follow steps for both men and women on how to come along side each other and helps you see the powerful effect working together can have. Leading a man to oils is simple, you just have to know how to do it! This will be a great tool for both men and women.

Grace Schlabach
Young Living Silver

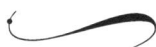

"You love your oils. You love your Husband. Your husband loves you, but may be baffled by your love of oils. Ron's book bridges the gap between Oils, Men & Women to figure it all out & find a way to love getting oily together and even have some fun along the way.

Ron's "Tales From The Oils Side" and quick wit give us insights into the male perspective and just how easy it really can be to overcome reluctance & resistance from the men in our lives & get them to hop onboard the oily train and join us on our oily journey.

What a blessing it is when we have our men who actually "get it" supporting & sharing about the oils right by our sides. Gratitude overflows thinking of the many women who have husbands, brothers, uncles, cousins

& friends who may find the tips in this book helpful for their own journey & bring health & abundance to so many more homes."

Colleen Holder
Young Living Silver

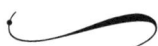

This book is EVERYTHING! It is wit and humor with a splash of serious talk for guys. Just what the Oily community needs. For all those guys out there that are skeptics, just put some peppermint on and watch the magic happen. For you ladies frustrated that your significant other might not be on board, give them this book! Ron does an incredible job laying it all out with simple explanations and practical tips.

Jodie Meschuk, founder @the.oil.vibe
Young Living Crown Diamond

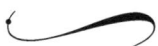

You Can Lead A Man To Oils....Takes the reader on a powerful journey into a woman's world of aromatherapy. This book is a guide for a specific kind of newly evolving man. Until fairly recently, modern roles for men and women were fixed and separated. Women were supposed to stay home and take care of the children. Men were supposed to go out and earn money. Chances are, if you are reading this book, you are more balanced than your parents were and you are in a relationship where little bottles of essential oils are showing up! This book is for men who choose to understand women, be it their lovers, mothers, daughters, or any other woman they interact with in their lives. Both men & women will gain insight into improving their relationships.

Ron's vulnerability and authenticity in sharing himself and his stories give us a new perspective into man's view. Through our life experiences we often come to know ourselves deeply through the heart of someone who loves us, who is willing to listen and engage. As uncomfortable as change can be, so many times it reveals the path to destiny. To have the quality of life and career success you desire, you'll have to roll up your sleeves and change some of those old beliefs that no longer work-the habitual behaviors that limit your effectiveness, block your joy, and tarnish your dreams. By embracing little things that mean so much to the ones we love, we create a new level of connection and intimacy with the ones we love the most. Accepting full responsibility for our lives and choosing connection over separation and understanding over defense we create a life of joy and happiness and smell good too!

Marcella Vonn Harting, PhD
Young Living Royal Crown Diamond

YOU CAN LEAD A MAN TO OILS...

You Can Lead a Man to Oils...

Your guide to understanding skeptical males

and motivating them to embrace essential oils

By Ron Corica

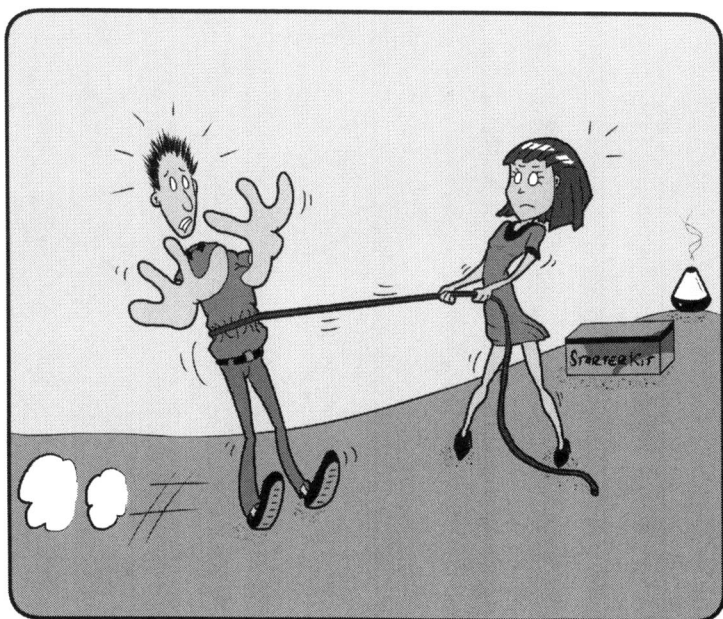

Disclaimer:
The concepts presented in this book are solely the perceptions and observations of the author. Young Living (or any other essential oil company) has not officially endorsed its contents, and neither are the views expressed in any way affiliated with Young Living. These personal statements should not be construed in any way as claims made by Young Living. The information contained in this book and the products mentioned are not meant to diagnose, treat, cure, or prevent any disease. Accordingly, the information presented represents what the author and other contributors experienced and observed through the usage of Young Living products. I am not a medical expert. Statements in this book have not been evaluated by the Food and Drug Administration.

Information found in this book is meant for educational and informational purposes only. The author desires to motivate you to make your own health-care and dietary decisions based upon your own continued research and in partnership with your health care provider. Use and application of this information is done solely at your own risk. Individual results may vary.

ISBN-13: 9781973836520
ISBN-10: 1973836521

All Scripture quotations, unless otherwise indicated, are taken from the Holy Bible: New American Standard. Copyright 1977 by the Lockman Foundation.

Oil Symphony Publications
Wentzville, MO 63385
oilsymphony@hotmail.com
www.yldist.com/oilsymphony

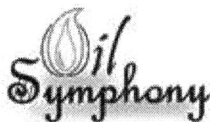

*To my wife, Diane, who led this resistant male
to oils with love, wisdom, and patience.
To my late father, Joe Corica. Before I knew
about oils, he was my "Valor."
To the glory of Jesus Christ.*

CONTENTS

ACKNOWLEDGMENTS

No undertaking of this sort is accomplished alone. Without the help, support, and encouragement from so many people, this book would not be a reality. Let me take a moment to name a few.

First, I need to thank my wife, Diane, for her constant encouragement, help, and support throughout this process. Evidently she loves me! At times, she alone was my "Stress Away." Diane kept me holding on to the bar during the emotional roller coaster of this project.

I would like to thank my son Daniel, whose illustrations and dedicated effort brought my ideas to life. The pictures helped to energize me along the way.

I'd like to thank author and friend Rhonda Rhea for letting me pick her brain and giving me insight into the process. She blessed me with her encouragement as well.

I am grateful to my in-laws, Don and Pat Horina, for putting up with my crazy ideas and wholeheartedly supporting this effort, particularly through their faithful prayers.

I would also like to give a shout out to those who contributed their personal stories. They bring clarity and depth to the text.

And in a wider scope, I'd like to say thanks to the members of the Oil Symphony, Oil Palooza, and Oil Vibe teams—and the Oil Vibe Dudes, too! The members share information so readily, encourage one another, and positively shaped our entry into this essential oil lifestyle.

DROP EVERYTHING!

I HAVE JUST RETURNED from attending my first Young Living annual convention. The 2017 convention was held in Salt Lake City, Utah. The setting was beautiful! Let me say it was an altogether enlightening and inspirational experience. It was exceptional not only for the many seminars and fantastic expo but also for my experience as it relates to this book.

The first morning, as I walked from the parking garage to the Salt Palace, a woman outpacing our group suddenly turned to me and thanked me for attending the convention. She said it was normal to see thousands of women in attendance, but not many men seemed concerned enough about their health. It actually encouraged her that I was there. What an introduction! It's not like I was the only guy there, but it was providential that she spoke those words to me, since I was writing this book.

That scene was repeated many times over the next three days. So many women related to me in similar words how wonderful it was to see men in attendance. Many also expressed frustration about their men, who wouldn't attend or use oils at all. Having random women volunteer their heartfelt feelings to a man they didn't know seemed strange to me at first. In time, I learned to embrace my new celebrity status. I began to stride into those seminars like a boss! I hadn't done anything epic or new; I was just ahead of the curve because I used essential oils and was present at the convention to carry my wife's backpack!

My desire to address this subject overwhelmed me at times as I walked through a sea of women, knowing that they were hurting. They were smiling on the out-side, yet inside there was this ever-present longing for their husbands to be present and supportive. I had already begun work on this book before leaving for the convention, realizing this irrational, reluctant male issue was apparent even among those on my wife's oil team. My convention experiences awakened me to the extent to which this male syndrome exists. This is my story as much as it is every man's story. Even more significantly, this is a story every essential oil-using woman can relate to. Either her husband is resisting or someone on her team has a reluctant male.

With renewed vigor I determined to complete this book to give women hope and encouragement. If you are a woman reading this book, chances are you already know the significance that a drop of oil can have in all kinds of applications. The hard part is—or in some cases, *was*—leading your man to oils and getting him to use them. By approaching this subject from a lighthearted angle, I hope you can relax, enjoy a few laughs, and be refreshed. I also want to challenge men to make wise choices about essential oil use and be heroes in their own families. I am anticipating great results once you let your man read this book, and he also learns to...drop everything!

Chapter 1

It's a "Woman" Thing!

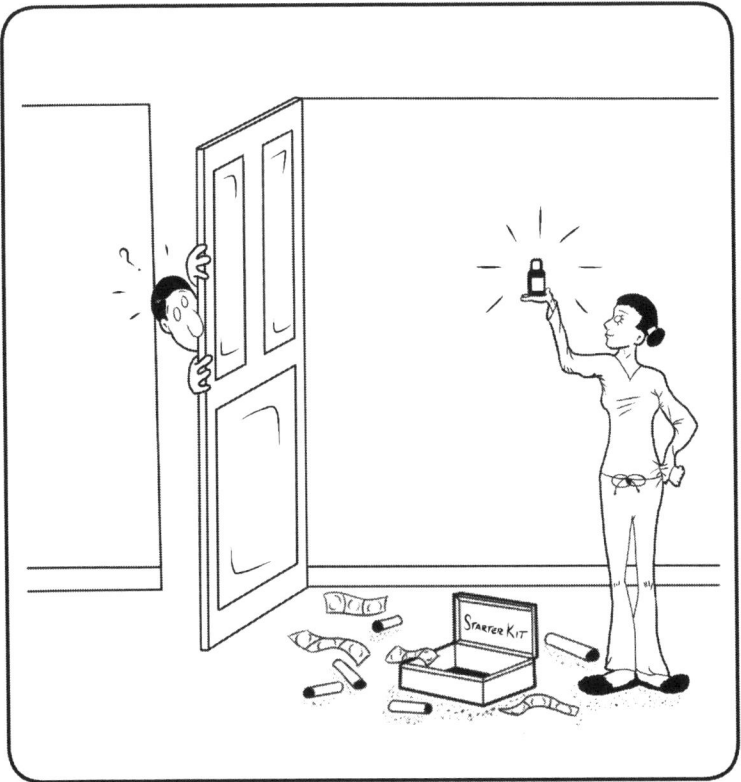

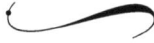

"He who restrains his words has knowledge, And he who has a cool spirit is a
man of understanding."

—*PROVERBS 17:27*

"He who speaks truth tells what is right,
But a false witness, deceit."

—*PROVERBS 12:17*

"And you shall know the truth, and the
truth shall make you free."

—*JOHN 8:32*

"If we are to better the future, we must
disturb the present."

—*CATHERINE BOOTH*

"My formula for success is rise early, work late and strike oil."

—J. PAUL GETTY

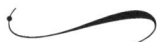

1

IT'S A "WOMAN" THING!

MY WIFE SPENT a solid hour putting Jewel, her part Arabian sorrel horse, through another training session. Walk, trot, lope. First moving in a clockwise direction around the arena before changing direction. Go around the barrels. Step over the poles. The many repetitions make it all look effortless. Around and around the practice continues. In late July the air gets stifling hot in the indoor arena and quite dusty. My job, besides stall cleaner and observer (supplying an authoritative "that looks good" at precisely the right moment), is to provide water to this hot, sweaty horse. But many of you know the old adage, "You can lead a horse to water, but you can't make him drink." No matter how hot the horse looked, and no matter how close I put the bucket of cool, refreshing water, I could not make her drink. Drinking the water had to be her idea. She might stand over it, sniff it, or nudge the bucket with her nose, but never actually drink the water. How frustrating that was for me, knowing the value that water could have for the horse. If she would only just take a sip!

Similar frustration is being experienced all over our country, maybe even the world, by women who cannot seem to get their men to use essential oils. There have been some awkward conversations and some pensive whiffs, but no regular buy-in. This reluctance of men to use oils is not just the unique experience of a few well-meaning women, anxious to see their husbands benefit from essential oil use. Amazingly, this appears to be widespread reality! Do a simple Google search for men and oils, and you will be amazed by what you see. There are many blogs that point out how women are more frequent users of essential oils than men. One such blog labels this divide between women and men's usage of oils as the "Fred Flintstone phenomenon" because men are so reluctant to try them. Other blogs pay homage to the "men don't use oils" sentiment by beginning their blog or article with a sentence about how hard it is to get a man "on board" with essential oils. A November 1, 2015, article in the *Men's Fitness* magazine was titled "Real Men Use

Essential Oils" in a peer-pressured attempt to tell men it is okay to use them. Once again, you can lead a man to oils...Many men will ignore, avoid, stall, dodge, and even *run* from a tiny application of essential oils. Unfortunately, I'm afraid this is the case with men for any product or event they deem is only for women. I'm not exactly sure how something gets a "for women only" designation, but the following story explains one way this can occur.

When my children were younger, my daughter began riding horses. It seemed many at the ranch where she took lessons were girls, probably a twelve-to-one ratio. When we tried to bring our boys for a fun day of riding, it was like pulling teeth. The suggestion was met with moans and groans and much rolling of the eyes. With four boys, that was a lot of eye rolling. Why, you may ask...bad weather? No. Was it the wildness of the horses? No. Was it the poor John Wayne impressions I was usually attempting—well, maybe that was part of it. But the overwhelming reason the boys did not want to participate was simply that "riding is for girls!" The perception of their sister doing this first, in a place where there were mostly girls, eventually became their reality.

I recognize that there are some things that actually have an appropriate "for women only" designation.

Pride and Prejudice and the *Home Shopping Network* come to mind. But it would be a shame to let essential oil use fall into the same category. The following is a case in point involving the "for women only" approach to essential oils.

I was at a social event and was introduced to a couple. The man noted that they had heard my wife speak at someone's in-home oil class. I was surprised that he was present at the class, but I was pleased he brought this up and assumed he had some lasting interest in the topic, so I pursued. He remembered that she talked about my story of introduction into oils, so I took the opportunity to retell my story firsthand. As we stood in line, waiting to get our finger food, I casually asked him what he thought of the oil presentation. Without hesitation, he shook his head and mumbled something about not caring about oils. In a sort of disbelieving tone, I asked a second time, figuring there was something redeeming about what he learned, but he simply responded, "Oils are for women." And with that we grabbed our egg-salad sandwiches and parted. I was disappointed with his response, as I had just told him my man-oil story! Once again, I remind you that this book is aimed at exploring this irrational, yet common, theme among men. I realize I live in the Show-Me state, so it may be particularly difficult for men here to get past the "oils are for women" mentality. We seem to need extra prodding, poking, and pushing before we are convinced. While you may live in an area where men are more easily convinced, I have discovered enough similarities around the country to realize the epic proportions of this male dilemma.

The following pages are provided to take a realistic look at the culture behind this phenomenon and some practical ways to address it. My aim is to make you laugh a little, think a lot, and accomplish even more. I hope to end the cycle of frustration for so many women and help men feel comfortable using essential oils and, dare I think it, even embrace a healthy lifestyle.

If you are just discovering essential oils, you may be asking yourself, "Why are these oils causing such a stir?" Here are some foundational thoughts to keep in mind as you go through the rest of this book. Essential oils are extracted from flowers, shrubs, trees, roots, bushes, resins, seeds, and other plants. They are considered volatile oils, because their scent molecules disperse quickly into the air. Inside the botanicals there is a flow of essential oils that carry nutrients throughout the plant to keep it alive and healthy. These oils are extracted through a distillation process. The energy frequencies of the oils produced correspond to the frequencies in a person's body. These pure, potent, therapeutic grade oils help support all the systems of the body. There are hundreds of various oils that affect a wide range of wellness issues. If you haven't already begun using them, don't let the oil train leave the station without you on it. You will then be exposed to an exciting new life!

In my neck of the woods, the culture of essential oils looks something like this: A woman has discovered essential oils. She talks about them with other women with excited laughter and gleeful expressions. Next, other women are encouraged to host informational gatherings or classes. Women of all ages attend, seeking help with physical, emotional, and even spiritual issues. Women invite other women. Many of these women begin to tout the wonderful fragrances in the colorful little bottles. The ladies relate the stories of these feminine gatherings to their husbands and families. They joyfully report the success stories of how women found help clearing up their skin or balancing hormones or simply sleeping better. That is certainly not a sequence that will send a man running to purchase and use the oils.

In the early days of my wife's essential oil use, she would frequently produce a bottle of an unknown substance, hold it under my nose, and ask, "Doesn't it smell good?" Now, to be honest, in some cases the fragrance smelled great! In other cases, I had to wonder what died in order to produce such a potion. This is an important point in the cultural issues between men and women. Women are all about fragrances. Whatever else an oil is or affects, it is first introduced as a fragrance. A man, however, does not live in a world of rose petals and lemon cleaner. He is comfortable with items that appear macho. Men don't typically gravitate toward the dainty or floral. Fragrance is not a chief selling point unless you are talking about food. Consider that motor oil doesn't "smell good," but men get smeared up to their elbows in it and seem to enjoy it. In this same vein, modesty prevents me from mentioning the gross things men apply to their bodies in preparation for a hunting trip. After all, if you can smell like a deer or bear, you have a better chance of getting one. It's not likely your man is out hunting for cinnamon or lavender.

A second factor in the culture surrounding essential oils involves listening. Women by far are better listeners. Through a woman's daily routine, she is remarkably prepared to pay attention to many things at once. While refereeing the children as they prepare for school, a busy mother can hear the pet's requests to go outside, log away her husband's supper plans, notice the washing machine has stopped, and all the while be watching a Young Living Diamond class on Facebook live. All that training makes a woman crave the nuances of oily information. There is a distinct intensity to a gathering of women at an oils class as they gobble up every juicy morsel of information they can.

On the flip side, many polls have shown that from a woman's perspective, men are poor listeners. This has been an issue that gets rehashed regularly over the years. One recent study was published in a February 25, 2016, issue of *Psychology Today*. Dr. Audrey Nelson asked more than one thousand people to identify gender strengths and weaknesses in communication. The women's number-one criticism of men was that they are "lousy listeners." Interestingly enough, the men agreed. An additional critique was that men sometimes "don't even make an effort to pretend they are listening..." So whether fact or perception, a man's listening deficiency has been a long-standing issue.

Often myopic in their attention, men struggle to focus on more than one thing at a time. Occasionally, you may find some men who are a little better at listening. Representing the other extreme, there are some men that are a few clowns short of a circus. They cannot seem to focus, period. On several occasions in my own experience, one or several of my children have stood next to me saying, "Dad…Dad…Dad…Father… Father Ron…" and in some astounding fashion I awaken from my stupor to finally acknowledge their pleas. Laughably, I felt quite noble that I was investing time with my children. Oh, the humanity! If you want to get rich, invent a device for the listening impaired.

All this to say, ladies…he's not listening! The entire time you are sparkling with exciting information about your recent oil class or latest product discovery, he's not listening. Oh, don't get me wrong; he may be looking directly at you, making eye contact, and even giving an occasional grunt of approval, but he is not really listening. It may appear frightfully close to a scene from *The Walking Dead*. His interest level is low, so the hardwired listening attachment in his gray matter is not activated. All of that essential oil "woman" stuff is barely a blip on his radar. To make matters worse, he probably doesn't care, either. In some strange way, men see essential oils and the accompanying lifestyle as a threat to their masculinity. With that as the backdrop, men don't care to know more, and neither do they want to get involved in this apparently feminine pastime. It really boils down to the question, "Does he want to listen?" I am not excusing this male flaw, just trying to be transparent about how things really are. After all, men *can* listen when they want to. Just ask the first men on the moon if they were listening to the instructions for getting back!

Contributing to the perception that oils are for women is the oily vernacular. This might be a partial solution to the problem of "he is not listening." It is not so much that the jargon is womanly, but it is decidedly not manly. There is little that would draw a man in or compel him to investigate. Deciding what "manly" speech is would be a difficult task, to be sure. Maybe it would serve our purpose to suggest areas of change that could help, instead of targeting specific words.

You may have noticed that men use a lot of acronyms. NFL, NHL, NASCAR, and NASA come to mind. IRS comes to mind, too, but I'd rather put that out of my mind, thank you. As drawing men in is the goal, a few prominent acronyms would help. You have to be well into your oil journey to discover PV and OGV, and those are not very compelling. Compelling to a man would be something like "OORAH"—Official Oils Reduce Archaic Hesitancy. How about "BOMB"— Basic Oils Manufactured Better...? With this acronym, men could truly say "These oils are the BOMB!"

If there was an acronym like "SPORT"—Scientifically Proven Oils Replace Tragedy," you would certainly get a man's attention. And what better way to win him over than with "FOOD"—Frequently Obtain Oil Drops!

Along with the creation of some manly acronyms, grabbing a man's interest would also be enhanced by some masculine phraseology. Ladies, instead of talking to him like you were talking to a group of women, try, "You need to use essential oils to enhance the body's machinery." Play on the fact that men love power tools and heavy equipment. You could say things that relate to a man's world like, "Using these oils will give you energy like a Monster Truck." It is well known that men thrive on fixing things. Use that to positively influence him toward oils. "The starter kit is a toolbox to fix what ails you." Do you see the huge difference in man-targeted speech versus normal woman lingo like, "These bottles are so cute and colorful"? Yeah, that will pique a man's interest. (Not!) You may not say that directly to him, but when he hears you say that to another woman, he checks out. If your goal is to convince a man, you have to try at least a little to think like one.

Let's not let the women off the hook here totally about this skewed oil perception. It seems women are complicit in spreading this false idea that "oils are for women." Realizing that the angelic realm is trembling at the notion that I would implicate the women in this sinister plot, I want you, ladies, to consider your actions and how they feed the false narrative. When you are first informed about essential oils or when you are invited to a class, not many women respond with something like, "I can't wait to tell my husband about this health option" or "I'll get my husband to come, too!" It is rather something a little closer to rounding up all your girlfriends, daughters, or mom to tell them about your new discovery. As oils are about health and wellness and not some New Age potion or fad, why does the husband, the father, or the sons seem to automatically get left out? When invitations are mailed out for upcoming oil events, why is the lady's name alone on the invitation? Why not invite the husband and wife to attend as a couple? Women who use oils and want to share the experience mostly talk to other women and take a backdoor approach to getting information to the men. In many cases, it is the women who make essential oils a "woman's" thing before it ever has a chance to be a man's thing.

The following account is a good example of the essential oil culture as described above. This was reported by Josh O'Meara in California:

My wife went to Hawaii on a yoga retreat, leaving me with the kiddos and these mystery liquids she brought home. She left me with a few tiny sample bottles of Lemon, Lavender, and Peppermint. I had no clue what to use them for.

At any rate, fast forward a day or two. My daughter was having a severe allergic reaction to something. Her hands were blazing red! I was freaking out, not knowing what to do. I was about ready to take her to the ER because she was very uncomfortable and crying. Finally, my wife responded to my frantic texts, "LLP baby, LLP." Outcome—no explanation needed!

Needless to say, it took a freaked-out dad with no clue what to do, and I became a believer."

Notice the terminology describing his involvement with the oils. He had "no clue," and he didn't know what to do with the oils. To this point it was just a "woman's thing" to Josh. I especially like the use of the term "mystery liquids." The oils are known to women, but the guys are in the dark. The women reach a comfort level using the oils long before many men do. For most men, essential oils are first perceived as mystery liquids for women. In the next chapter, we will see what encourages guys to have many imaginative thoughts about these mystery snake oils.

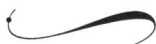

THE LAST DROP

Ok, ladies! It's time to change the perception of essential oils. I challenge you to find ways to get men involved in the process. Have couples' classes. Invite a man to present your 101 class or some other topic. Be creative. After all, you don't really believe that it's a "woman's thing," do you?

Guys, if you're still thinking oils are for women, *stop*! Oils are about wellness. You can enter in, and it does not have to be weird. Women do a lot of the cooking, but men eat, right? Men do not starve themselves just because cooking is a "woman thing." (If you do, we need to have a serious talk.) Dig a little deeper past that feminine first impression. You will be glad that you did.

"How many men does it take to screw in a light bulb? One—he just holds it up there and waits for the world to revolve around him."

—A<small>NONYMOUS</small>

"Stressed spelled backwards is desserts!"

—A<small>NONYMOUS</small>

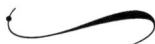

Chapter 2

What Is This New Age, Voodoo, Hippie Stuff?

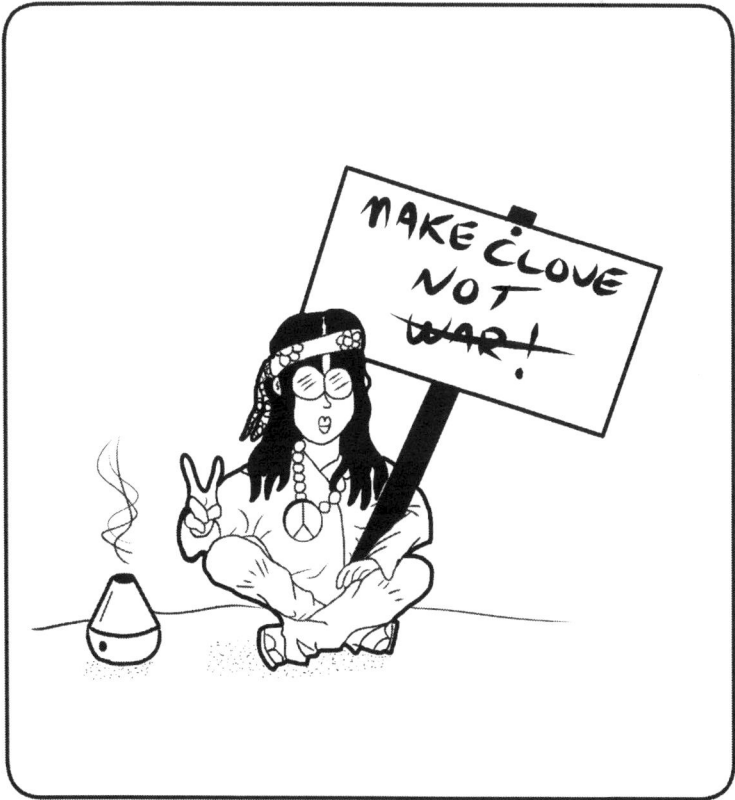

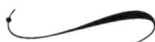

"Thou dost prepare a table before me in the presence of my enemies; Thou hast anointed my head with oil; My cup overflows."

—PSALM *23:5*

"Let your clothes be white all the time, and let not oil be lacking on your head."

—ECCLESIASTES *9:8*

"A keen sense of humor helps to overlook the unbecoming, understand the unconventional, tolerate the unpleasant, overcome the unexpected and outlast the unbearable."

—BILLY GRAHAM

"Learn from the mistakes of others. You can't live long enough to make them all yourself."

—ELEANOR ROOSEVELT

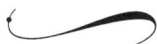

2

WHAT IS THIS NEW AGE, VOODOO, HIPPIE STUFF?

COULD MY WIFE be having a midlife crisis? What in the world are these crazy concoctions she's making? Has my wife been secretly watching some Internet guru who has masterfully convinced her that the hippie movement is not dead? All of this is "far out, man." At times I catch her applying scented oils to various body parts. She has curiously added walking around with necklaces and bracelets that ooze greenhouse gasses. And then there are the dimly lit diffusers with exotic fragrances wafting through the house during the day and in the bedroom as we sleep. My wife's morning ritual now includes applying some oils on a regular basis. In fact, she has begun to drop everything. No, not literally dropping items on the floor. She's now applying drops of oil on everything for every reason.

Once in a while, she will throw in a random "snake oil" she splashes on to address specific health issues at various times of the day. Then there are the women's classes that meet like a secret society, generating a cult-like following among the users. What else goes on at these "classes"? Does someone play the bongos and read poetry? Next thing you know, there will be beads hanging up around the house and neon orange shag carpeting splashed across the living-room floor. Worse yet, she may ask to move to some commune. By the way, how is all this related to wellness? What ever happened to aspirin and chicken soup? For that matter, what ever happened to my wife?

Ladies, if you have ever wondered what your man is thinking when he is hiding in the other room, wonder no more! While you are chuckling over your husband's wild imagination and harebrained thought life, try to understand his point of view. Many of these masculine thoughts are rooted in an honest perception of the transformation taking place within his own home and, even more threatening, within his own wife! Men are more inclined to be skeptical because they were created to be protectors. When things appear different or strange, a man's antenna goes up, and he is on the lookout for danger or trickery. Of course, it could be that men simply have a much thicker blood-brain barrier for oils to pass through, and that is why it takes men much longer to catch on. The reasons women buy and use essential oils vary greatly, but women gravitate toward them more quickly than men. In general, men tend to be skeptical observers only. To the men this is all some kind of blast from the past but with no current merit.

If you recall, the hippie movement of the 1960s and 1970s had many components that seem similar to an oily lifestyle. Let's do a quick comparison of the two. Part of the hippie scene involved getting back to nature, certainly in things that they ate, but also in what they wore and what they rejected. In fact, I'm expecting Young Living to release a new product line at a coming convention—YL Bell bottoms! But I digress. Let's stick to the food for now. Young Living can also revive a slogan for their many consumable items, "Don't panic, it's organic!" Those desiring organic products were labeled as "countercultural" at that time. Today, there is a discernable similarity to the ideals of the past with the growing attention on organically grown foods and natural remedies. This natural approach to food and wellness is apparent with many essential oil users as well.

Many people today are uninformed about the food they eat. Allow me to "lay some thoughts on you."

The food is accepted because it's assumed it is vetted by the grocery store. If you are brave enough to do a little digging, you can uncover many facts about the food we purchase so readily. The processing of foods depletes them of nutrition. The widespread use of chemicals, pesticides, and GMOs on products that eventually make it to the store shelf warrant counter-culture action. We used to wash a piece of fruit before eating it to get the dangerous junk off the outside. With the enormous use of chemicals the plant or tree absorbs from the ground, the dangerous junk is now *in* the fruit as well as *on* it. The plant itself may be genetically modified, so you don't know for sure what you are getting and the effect it will have on you. The tiny, "acceptable" amounts of poison in each portion are all adding up to unacceptable health complications. The American Cancer Society has addressed these very issues in a website article dated January 11, 2012, and revised in February 2016. The article, entitled "Food Additives, Safety and Organic Foods," reviews these same issues as they apply to cancer risk. Their conclusions are very "uncool." One statement reads, "Unintended contamination of food may also result in exposure to chemicals that are a cause of concern and may be related to cancer risk. Examples include heavy metals such as cadmium or mercury." These are not advertising headlines the food industry wants you to be aware of. This is why it is imperative to do your own research. So yeah, a little countermeasure is needed. I never thought I would like being called a "nonconformist," but it is actually quite exhilarating!

Another similarity to past hippie culture, which confuses the oil observer, is doing things that go against the established norms. Today, those who boldly venture into systematic essential oil usage are spearheading the effort to break away from the accepted medical practices and prescriptions of our day and blaze a new trail towards wellness. The side effects of many of the drugs are outrageous. Oils help you avoid them. Staying healthy is more advantageous than having to fix chronic health issues. The amount of unnecessary surgeries performed these days is another reason to stay healthy and break from current norms. *USA Today* exposed this assault on the innocent in their June 19, 2013, article by Peter Eisler and Barbara Hansen. The caption under the title reads, "A *USA Today* study found that tens of thousands of times each year, patients undergo surgeries they don't need." Wow, that will blow your mind! I don't know about you, but I would like to keep all my parts as long as possible.

The use of incense in homes and clubs to encourage the right atmosphere was at one time a fashionable part of the hippie culture. In essential oil households and offices, there are diffusers strategically placed for both aesthetic and health reasons. The oils don't just smell good; they can inject calmness or clarity into the atmosphere and so much more. Let me hear you say, "Groovy, man!" For the male skeptic, this is another reason to be wary of the oils. The oil fragrances being diffused throughout the house seem like a time-warp to him. More recently, the New Age movement has likewise used incense diffusers, focused on natural food and health and finding energy from the earth. Unfortunately, there may be too much emphasis on the earth itself, and not enough emphasis on the Creator. Those distortions cause skepticism about natural oils and their by-products. So why are the women so committed even if the men remain skeptical?

For many women, the use of essential oils was fueled by a widespread search for wellness options. Those options may have included eating healthier, detoxifying their homes from harmful chemicals, or finding natural alternatives to the complicated side effects that accompany pharmaceuticals. While this bonanza of natural help through essential oils is gratifying to a woman, once again you must consider a male perspective. A home under the influence of an essential oil user morphs into a new place over time. Oil bottles are strategically placed throughout the house, on sinks, in various drawers, and on nightstands. Reference books and support books begin to pile up on the desk and maybe on the floor. Cardboard tubes multiply like rabbits. (BTW, guys—these make good fire starters in the winter!) Hand soaps are missing from the sinks. Laundry detergent is being homemade instead of store-bought. An oil-infused drink of water has to be from a stainless steel or glass container. Spritzers and sprayers are nestled all over the house. The husband finds himself being given new instructions about eating and cleaning, sometimes on a daily basis. I have had to slip away to the basement on several occasions to scarf down a Ding Dong in secret in order to avoid incurring another health lecture.

While that just scratches the surface of changes that may be taking place in the home, consider the many changes taking place in (and to) the wife. Gone from her routine are the hair sprays and harsh skin cleaning chemicals she previously used. In some cases, makeup is being replaced or rejected all together. Oils of one kind or another are being applied for one reason or another as part of her daily preparation. Sometimes the oils go on without a specific reason. The bottle just happened to be close. At night, there is an evening oil application ritual before retiring. In the morning there is a similar ritual. This ritual features oil applications and a red potion, which is some kind of oil-infused drink to energize the start of the day. As the need arises throughout the day, oils are being randomly applied or diffused, all of which may seem a bit "far out" to a man.

The funky word games are another one of those peculiar essential oil user quirks that keep the mystery wheel turning. It seems that in order to use essential oils, a new vocabulary must be acquired. Back in the 1960s, the hippie crowd had its own "outta sight" vocabulary too. I noticed my wife was often beating around the bush instead of telling me straight up what she was using an oil for or what it was intended to help fix. You know what I'm talking about, ladies… the dreaded compliance issue. When I was an oil novice and agreed to attend my wife's class for the first time, I was confused by the jumbled speech and the rephrasing of things. You know, the indirect way you try to direct people without being direct! All this altered speech is, in reality, an attempt to be compliant. This guarded speech, however, can cast a shadow of suspicion on the oil guild. I thought, *This is Weirdsville!* I took a peek outside to see if a flower-painted Volkswagen Bug was parked there. When I finally understood something clearly, that was when she would say, "I probably shouldn't have said that." Go figure! It took a while, but in time I learned the new lingo such as "help support," "assist body systems," "not intended to…," or "eases severe head tension." Groovy, man!

This is not to say involvement in essential oils is some sort of out-of-time hippie movement. I am just relaying the musings of an awkward first impression that is common among men. Oils are not connected to New Age theology, and neither is essential oil participation some sort of weird voodoo ritual. The local witchdoctor has not concocted the potions you are investing in. In reality, there is nothing strange, suspect, or shady about the production and application of essential oils. Although perception of the many changes in home products, food, and speech may be skewed, essential oil usage is based on a long history, solid science, and modern technologies.

Consider the fact that the oils come from plants created by God. The energy in the plant is put there by God. It was no mistake that God created Adam and Eve and placed them in a garden where they were exposed to plant oils and aromatherapy from the start. He even put them there in bare feet! They were soaking in oily goodness even when they did not know it. God intended oils to heal and bless, so why should we be so squeamish when someone actually uses them? Though oils were a known commodity for thousands of years, they slipped into the background during the modern era, particularly in North America. We had drifted away from their regular use over time. Essential oils are now making a resounding comeback! Modern harvesting innovations, distilling techniques, and quality control measuring devices create a super product for the twenty-first century. Oils legitimately deliver wellness support through a reliable, ancient product that may bewilder the uninitiated. And the beat goes on...

With all of that in mind, a man would be living in oblivion to not notice the changes—and not wonder, at least a little, what is happening to his wife and his household. No, these pure, potent products do not have any ties to witchcraft or voodoo or any other bizarre practice. The natural force in essential oils that assist healing in the body and ease the emotions is nothing weird or spooky. It is only that we have moved so far from the use of natural products and home remedies that it just seems out of place. Our society is now very comfortable with all things chemical, artificial, institutional, and mechanical.

You can expect to get some crazy looks, snubs, and weird misconceptions when you begin using essential oils. People, including husbands, tend to react when something is outside the realm of "normal." In our day of prim and proper subdivisions and homeowner associations, try hanging laundry outside to dry, and see if you get a strange reaction from your neighbors! Seeing people's underwear dangling on a line is no longer normal.

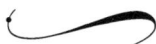

THE LAST DROP

Ladies, realize there will be some strange associations made with your involvement in essential oils. Do not let that worry or frustrate you. Instead, enjoy the ride. Stay cool. Being cheerful will override misconceptions and attract others.

Guys, don't get uptight. Your wife is not a hippie, and she did not join a cult. Cut her some slack. While your home life may seem a bit different, the changes that are happening are for the good. Embrace them. While you're at it, embrace her!

"A foolish man tells his wife to stop talking,
but a wise man tells her that her mouth is
extremely beautiful when her lips are closed."

—ANONYMOUS

"Some days I amaze myself! Other days I put
the laundry in the oven."

—ANONYMOUS

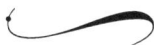

Chapter 3

Not Another Fad

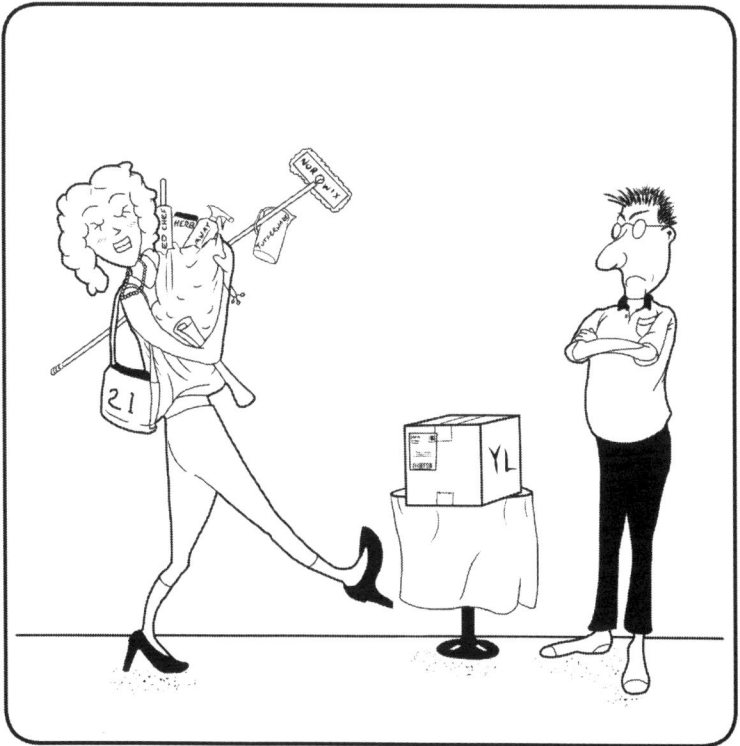

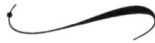

"Then the LORD said to Moses, "Take for yourself spices, stacte and onycha and galbanum, spices with pure frankincense; there shall be an equal part of each."

—E*XODUS* 30:34

"And they came into the house and saw the Child with Mary His mother; and they fell down and worshiped Him; and opening their treasures they presented to Him gifts of gold and frankincense and myrrh."

—M*ATTHEW* 2:11

"Nothing is more obstinate than a fashionable consensus."

—M*ARGARET* T*HATCHER*

"Even if you're on the right track, you'll get run over if you just sit there!"

—*WILL ROGERS*

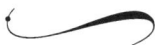

3

NOT ANOTHER FAD

Now, WHAT FAD has my wife been sucked into? What wonder product has swept my wife off her feet for the next few months? What is it that she has "just gotta have today"? These are normal questions for the average man to ask. First, it was beauty products. Next, she had to have the Rachel Green hairstyle like all of her, um, friends. After we had children, it was selling books. The next greatest thing was parties that displayed kitchen gadgets. Then the craze was baskets, vitamins, and now oils. "Rub some on," she says, "and be amazed!" Oh, I'm amazed all right! I'm amazed that she has found another fad to latch onto. Or *is* it another fad?

Women seem to find new fads to get excited about faster than gossip travels around an office party. The allure of "new," "chic," "easy," and "fast" captivates a woman's imagination. The pull of being a part of the "in" crowd can be downright irresistible. Besides acquiring information or purchasing the latest, greatest products, the party atmosphere surrounding network marketing is fantastic. Think of it—a dozen women gathered together, getting their "girl" time, with all that "girl" talk. You know what I mean: "Hi, girlfriend!" "What's up, girl?" "That's right, girl!" "Girl, shut up!" "Aww, girl!" You go, girl!" and just *"Girl...!"* (I resist any further commentary.) In many cases no children are present, only large applications of makeup, flattery, and hormones. There are usually plenty of hugs to go around and finger foods to munch. The combination of all of these profoundly contributes to a woman's sense of belonging. As described earlier, essential oil gatherings have a similar appearance.

Now, to be fair, it is understood that interest in essential oils is growing. Health and wellness issues are extremely prominent today, thanks in part to the abundance of aging baby boomers and a younger generation awakening to health issues. I am not suggesting that anyone should consider essential oils a fad, least of all the women. In fact, we are reminded by the Bible verses that are quoted at the beginning of the chapter that Frankincense has been around for over four thousand years! The wise men also brought some Frankincense and Myrrh to Jesus two thousand years ago, so, no, it is not a fad. In fact, I am almost certain Darth Vader even implored young Luke Skywalker to give in to the power of the *drop* side. Granted, there is currently a rebirth of knowledge surrounding oils, and with that knowledge, there is a surge in current use. However, with the many new changes that are taking place in the homes of essential oil users and the similarities to familiar fads, understand that there may be some overlap in how it is perceived. Once again I give this reminder to consider all of this from a man's point of view.

Every decade seems to have its fads. They come and they go. The 1970s had disco music, pet rocks, and mineral supplements. The 1980s saw the advent of big hair, boom boxes, and kitchen gadgets. The 1990s whisked in beanie babies and fanny packs and herbal products. In the 2000s we witnessed the rise and fall of the Atkins diet and flash mobs. Now we are discussing essential oils. A man's initial perspective on all things essential oil-related sees only that it has all the trappings of past, quick hit fads. First, the women head out to join their friends at an oils "class." A woman may mention the class several times, but a man hears and thinks "party." When the women return home, they cheerfully inform their husbands of the grand time they had gabbing with the other ladies, the interesting pick food that was sampled, and the fun things they learned about the oils...they purchased. So why wouldn't men think that this is all part of the latest fad? After all, didn't their wives just get their latest handbags from such an event? "This too shall pass," he opines.

Truth be told, women most likely explain a lot more about the oils, including their fragrance and how they support a healthy lifestyle. But as the man nervously watches his college basketball team blow the lead in the final moments of a close game, he is not paying much attention to his wife's "party" report. He half-heartedly responds with a courteous "It sounds like a fun night," hoping that will suffice so he can resume watching his stress-inducing game. Meanwhile, the woman glides back to her room, satisfied with the update she gave that managed to keep the expense and commitment to her new oil passion out of the conversation. Several days later, the shipment of oils arrives by mail. It is assumed by the unsuspecting man that this is all a part of the silly oil craze and will eventually fade. The female, however, like an exuberant child waking early on Christmas morning, rips into the box with great fervor, and the oils and oily products are gleefully displayed and sampled. Every few weeks the scenario repeats itself. Some of the same oils are repurchased, but there are usually some new oils or products in the box that will generate as much excitement as box number one. New oils in the box mean new uses in the home. Out with the old, in with the new is the reigning pattern. Toxic, chemical-laden, petroleum-based products slowly begin to vanish, replaced by essential oils, blends of essential oils, or oil-infused products. The reluctant male's notion that essential oils are a fad begins to fade over time as well…But not without a fight!

The aforementioned replacement procedure most likely will be met with some resistance. Who wants to say good-bye to the beloved toothpaste they have used for thirty-plus years? Who can easily give up their favorite morning beverage or their old, reliable hand soap? What man wants to give up his upset stomach remedy, even if it does not actually work very well? After all, he has always taken care of his stomach pain that way. Maybe the hardest to part with is the medicine cabinet full of cut, scrape, and soreness remedies that you have grown accustomed to over a lifetime. The winds of change do eventually begin to blow harder, however, and the replacements become more frequent and more drastic.

For the woman routinely using essential oils, the changes are fascinating and welcome. She is feeling a sense of victory due to overcoming the toxic world while making herself and her family safer and healthier. For the man of the house, who is still in the dark about the use, value, and rewards of essential oils, the changes are outrageous! He struggles to maintain his own quantity of his toiletries and cleaning products. He may lash out occasionally about not having what he needs when he needs it. He may angrily proclaim that he is not a willing participant in all the changes. He may say the proverbial "These oils are for women" line to justify his dogmatism. Women, do not be overzealous about accelerating the changes. Remain patient. Like a paper towel absorbing a spill, he is slowly getting educated and acclimated to everyday usage of essential oils.

Check out this account from one of our team members in Florida. I'll venture a guess that it will ring true for many of you. Alicia Blunt says:

> Joe was reluctant to start using oils, like most men. I finally got him his own bottle of Peppermint to support digestion. We no longer use over the counter products for that... Yay! Now he is good about carrying his own

bottle and usage. In fact, I have even caught him sharing it with his buddies. I found out when I returned from a trip and talked to a friend of ours. He asked me what that oil was that Joe shared with him. I was like, "Are you sure it was MY JOE?" It was, in fact, my Joe, and he had shared the Peppermint I'd given him. His friend was having some stomach issues that lasted for days, and he said the Peppermint was the only thing that worked for him. Six months later, I catch Joe again. This time he was defending our oils to another set of friends on Facebook. These friends did not believe in the oils' potency and were giving oil users grief, so hubby stood up for us! What has happened to my Joe?! He is still not a huge oil user, but will ask me when he needs to resolve some health concern. I just introduce things slowly to him and stay consistent.

Bravo, Alicia and Joe! They have overcome the fad impression and are moving their oil journey forward. Rather than a fad that fades over time, oils are experiences that expand over time.

In many cases, assisting the changes taking place in the home are the children. While the husband is keeping up his resistance, children appear to embrace the changes far more readily. They are flexible with change, as any habits they have formed or any favorites they may claim are not deeply rooted. Experience has taught them that when Mom suggests something new, it usually works out pretty well. We'll make an exception for the whole "eat your peas" thing. Whether it is getting their own roller ball, oils rubbed on their feet, or getting to suck on a NingXia Red packet, children find the oily life enjoyable. The jubilant way children incorporate the oils into daily use, and the results that occur, drive the changes in the home more rapidly.

Eventually, as a toxin-free home takes root, the household members begin to realize that essential oils are not a fad but are, in fact, a lifestyle change. Maybe the words "lifestyle change" sound a little too drastic; however, that is the direction the tide of essential oil usage eventually takes you. While it is easy to equate essential oils to a simple fad at first, consider that essential oils have been helping people feel better and supporting healthier lives for thousands of years. The pendulum of health is swinging back from man-made products to natural, time-tested products. With the increase in use, education, and experimentation with essential oils, a lifestyle change is inevitable, given the wonderful results and proven track record. And don't worry—although oil usage is resurgent, disco is not making a comeback.

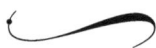

THE LAST DROP

Ladies, you are in this for the long haul. Essential oils have been doing their thing for a long time, and you should too. Lifestyle changes happen over time and with repetition. Keep consistency in what you are doing, and hubby will catch on in time.

Guys, your wife's use of essential oils will produce sweeping changes over time. Fads make a big splash, but lifestyle changes are like a river…it just keeps coming. Take heart in the fact that the changes are powerful and for everyone's good.

> *"It seems like Google must be a woman. It won't let you finish your sentence without coming up with another suggestion."*
>
> —*ANONYMOUS*

"I've had so much plastic surgery, when I die they will donate my body to Tupperware."

—JOAN RIVERS

"You never know what you have...until you clean your room!"

—ANONYMOUS

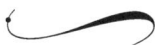

Chapter 4

The Dreaded Pyramid Scheme

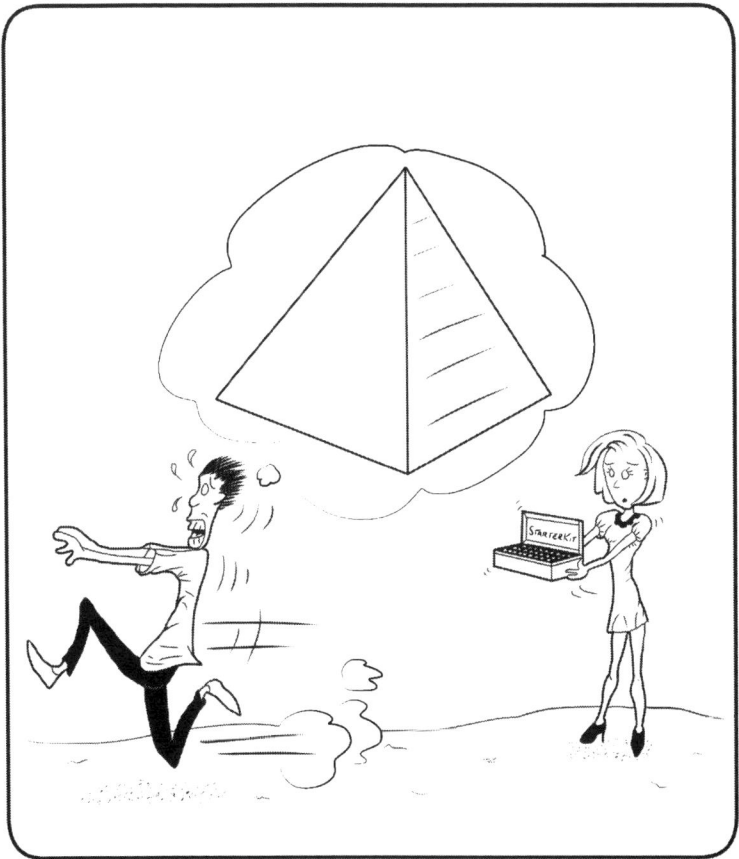

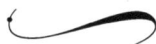

"The wages of the righteous is life, The income of the wicked, punishment."

—Proverbs 10:16

"The wicked earns deceptive wages, But he who sows righteousness gets a true reward."

—Proverbs 11:18

"If I would be given a chance to start all over again, I would choose Network Marketing."

—Bill Gates

"If you don't read the newspaper you're uninformed. If you do read the newspaper you're misinformed."

—Mark Twain

"When I tell any truth it is not for the sake of convincing those who do not know it, but for the sake of defending those who do."

—WILLIAM BLAKE (BRITISH POET)

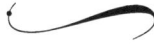

4

THE DREADED PYRAMID SCHEME

M Y POOR WIFE. She doesn't realize how she is being duped, taken in, hoodwinked! I must come to her aid and rescue her from this slippery slope. This can be the heartfelt responsibility awakened in a man upon first hearing of his wife's involvement in selling essential oils. We men are such skeptics. The football game we just watched was "fixed." The local mechanic is ripping us off. There is a conspiracy to make sure we catch all the red lights. Worldwide scams like "global warming" do not help in creating a trustworthy atmosphere. The sentiment is "You must remain vigilant or you will be snookered out of house and home at any moment."

The proverbial "red flag" that is swiftly hoisted to the top of the flagpole has less to do with the specific

YOU CAN LEAD A MAN TO OILS...

selling of essential oils and more to do with the concept of network marketing in general. Over the years, network marketing has fallen into the dirty basket along with the ever-frightful pyramid schemes. The bad connotations that have encrusted themselves to the pyramid scheme title have latched onto network marketing like a metastasizing cancer. This is an unfortunate association for those involved in network marketing.

There is a hilarious cartoon video posted to Youtube. com by Pat Petrini that captures the essence of this chapter by giving everyone a good laugh at the expense of those stubborn naysayers who hold onto their opinion no matter what facts are presented. In the video, one character is attempting to explain his desire to start his own network marketing business in order to get ahead financially and break away from the conventional work model. The second character stubbornly insists that it all sounds like a pyramid scheme. No matter how calmly and rationally network marketing is explained, the answer is always the same: "It sounds like a pyramid scheme." Facts are given, and influential financial people are even mentioned as backing this form of business, but to no avail. The second character is convinced that this is a pyramid scheme. This seems to be the case for many men when they hear about the businesses their wives are attempting to build.

Let me take a moment to explain the differences between network marketing and pyramid schemes.

Pyramid schemes engulf people on the promise of huge financial return for their initial financial investment into the company. If the salesman is good, a person is left seeing only dollar signs without asking very many in-depth questions. What makes it illegitimate is not the fantastic promise of fortune but rather the fact that there are no real goods or services being provided. Pyramid schemes are merely a shell game of taking funds, investing those funds, and moving the money around to provide dividend returns to investors. As long as more are investing than getting returns, the scheme is successful. Once the balance tips toward more people demanding payouts, the jig is up!

The exponential use of home computers spurred on network marketing in the 1990s and the years following. Many people found opportunities to create and grow a business right from home. A December 2000 article by Michael L. Sheffield, found on Entrepreneur.com, explains the legitimacy of network marketing. His first point is that in network marketing, people are being provided with "real, legitimate products" that people want and can use at reasonable prices. Because people have passion for their own businesses and excitement about their successful products, they grow financially mostly through their own elbow grease in sharing about the products and growing a sales team. In true network marketing, not only are products sold, but there is a premium put on education, personal development, and instruction, all of which enhance the value of being a part of the network organization.

Let's keep in mind that, in essence, every business has a "pyramid" structure. A bank has a president, several vice-presidents, many more managers and department heads, and then a layer of supervisors before you get to the operational workers carrying out the daily duties normally associated with banking, such as tellers and clerks. I have not heard people call the pyramid structure of a bank into question, because it provides a service people need. In much the same way, a retail store you may frequent has an owner, a CEO, many managers, and many more supervisors and workers. Once again, the products provided when you shop allow for acceptance of the pyramid structure of the local store. The grocery store has an owner, a few vice-presidents, several store managers, many supervisors, and many clerks—a pyramid structure, to be sure. Network marketing is legitimatized by its products as well, but unlike stores or banks, the network marketing format allows options for individuals to build a business, investing time as they can, with low overhead and unlimited geographical limitations. The supervisors and workers are not housed under one roof, but they are scattered in homes locally and possibly across the globe.

Separating network marketing of essential oils from any scheme is the supremacy that is placed on service to people. Pyramid schemes take advantage of people. As much as you love essential oils, it is imperative to keep in mind that people are the focus. Oils support wellness; people get well. Oils reach into the body systems; people inhabit those bodies. Oils can bring financial freedom; people enjoy that freedom. The oils themselves are not the end, but a means to an end. Use oils and love people and take great caution not to use people and love oils. Oils are simply tools. You may even call them "power" tools. These potent products are tools for connecting, for helping, for encouraging, and for strengthening people. Never neglect the person holding the bottle. People are to be loved and shown compassion. Great relationships can be built through network marketing. Oils are one of the tools that make that happen.

When a woman begins to talk about a network marketing oil business, many men want to flee. The work environment a man is in all day provides enough problems and pressures, so he does not quickly embrace more pressure at home. So what does he do? He avoids the conversation. Avoidance is a man's best defense. Have you ever noticed that when a discussion of essential oils begins, the man who was just lounging on the couch watching football becomes the busiest house-cleaning machine you ever saw? He instantly remembers the garage needs to be cleaned. Suddenly, doing the dishes is a great idea. Cleaning out the closet becomes a top priority. In the inner workings of most men, talking about subjects they don't know much about or that seem strange to them amounts to pressure. The best way to avoid pressure is to run from it. They become as good at escaping as Captain Jack Sparrow! Believe me when I say, not too many men want to do the dishes or clean their rooms. However, in the face of hearing tales from the oils side, even cleaning seems like a good idea. Learning details about oils is pressure. Learning new ways to apply the oils is pressure. Hearing about a myriad of women who use oils and why they use them is pressure. Being forced to use new products is pressure. All these new and incredible changes are pressure. A man imagining his wife is involved in a pyramid scheme is pressure. Trying to figure out how to graciously talk her out of it is even more pressure! At work, a person must lean in to the pressure and overcome it. At home, a man wants to simply escape pressure in any way he can.

As we are discussing alleviating pressure, it may be helpful at this point to give information on the compensation plan. Making money is a good thing. Making money helps reduce pressure. Making lots of money…well, you get the idea. Mentioning other successful and respected network marketing companies might help reduce pressure and skepticism as well. I do not know each individual situation of those reading this book. I will say, however, that this is a major obstacle for men. Why? Because before they know much about essential oils or the Young Living company, they will get a lot of negative feedback in this area. Many people default to the pyramid scheme mantra just because it is commonly discussed. It is easy for a man to get swept away in the negativity. But be encouraged. Your steady health improvements and growing paychecks will help him pay more attention to what you are telling him than what others say. There is power in your progress!

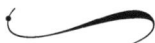

THE LAST DROP

Okay, ladies, take a deep breath. In through the nose...out through the mouth. This may be the hardest obstacle you will need to get your man over. The truth is freeing, so don't get bogged down with the negativity of others. Essential oils are impactful, and sharing about them in your business is rewarding.

Guys, I get the skepticism, but get over it already! Essential oils are legit! The business model is a proven one. Don't get hung up on old stereotypes. If you think about it, all businesses pay out more at the top than at the bottom. Encourage your wife as she works her way up. Don't fear the pyramid; use the network.

> *"A woman has the last word in any argument. Anything a man says after that is the beginning of a new argument!"*

—ANONYMOUS

> *"Hold your wife's hand in the mall. It looks romantic but it's actually economic. If you let go she'll start shopping."*

—ANONYMOUS

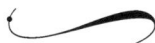

Chapter 5

Men Need Breathing...and Data

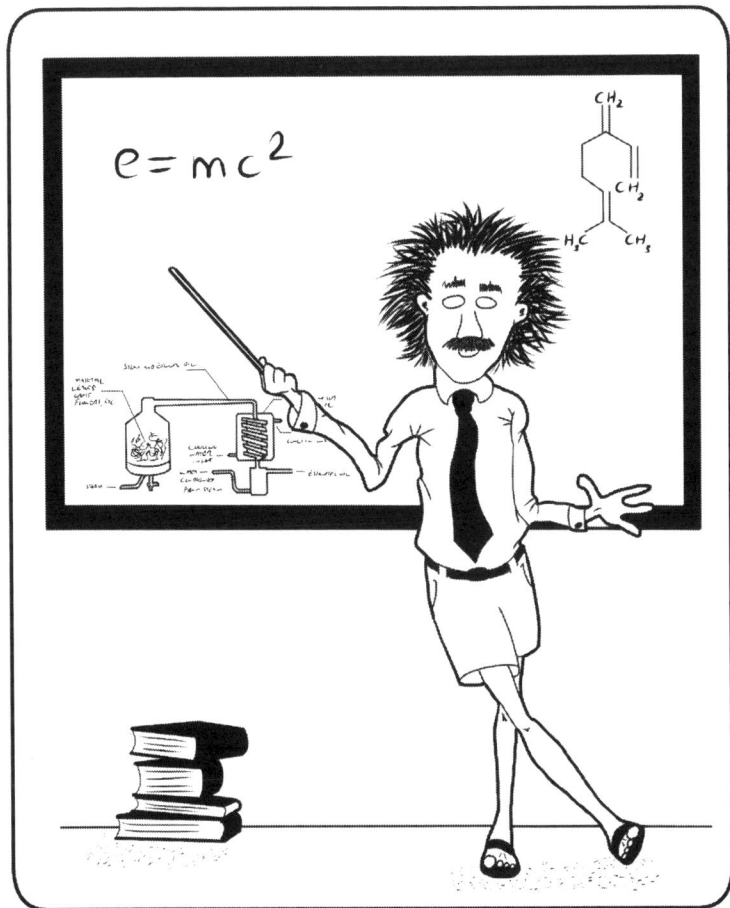

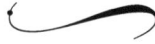

"How blessed is the man who finds wisdom, And the man who gains understanding."

—*PROVERBS 3:13*

"Heed instruction and be wise, And do not neglect it."

—*PROVERBS 8:33*

"The tongue of the wise makes knowl-edge acceptable…"

—*PROVERBS 15:2*

"Some of the best theorizing comes after collecting data because then you become aware of another reality."

—*ROBERT J. SHILLER (WINNER OF NOBEL PRIZE IN ECONOMICS)*

"Most of the world will make decisions by either guessing or using their gut. They will either be lucky or wrong."

—S*UHAIL* D*OSHI* (CEO, M*IXPANEL*)

"Don't let schooling interfere with your education."

—M*ARK* T*WAIN*

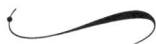

5

MEN NEED BREATHING...AND DATA

WITHOUT BREATHING, LIFE wouldn't be possible. Okay, so I'm stating the obvious. The rhythmic, life-producing inhaling and exhaling energizes the body systems without conscious perception. There are exceptions in cases where people overexert themselves and then pant like overheated puppies. Physical strain produces the need for more rapid and powerful air intake. What should be just as obvious is that a man's world revolves around data. In the same almost unconscious fashion, men are perpetually collecting and analyzing data. Data propels resolutions forward. Just like breathing, there is an increased need for solid data when tough decisions have to be made or important plans have to be executed. You can lead a man to essential oils, but you'll find it's a big leap to get him to use the oils without the proper data. Keep in mind, "They smell good" is not data. "They help with well-ness" is not data. Men want rock-solid, indisputable, numerical, spreadsheet data. Men seem to thrive when the detailed information is plentiful. Facts and fig-ures, procedures, and timetables are a dramatic part of both their work and their hobbies. "How many?" and "How often?" and "How come?" make up the stim-uli for gathering a myriad of data points, whether for business or pleasure. A man just cannot seem to make enough withdrawals from the data bank.

The data we are discussing is nothing more than organized information. Data fuels any worthwhile enterprise a man is about to embark on. In some ways, it is the preponderance of data that creates a man's love for sports. From batting averages, strike-out ratios, yards per carry, completion percentages, field-goal percentages, and even save percentages, the sports world is filled with data categories for men to sift through, compare, and argue about. Most of the information is called statistics but let's face it, statis-tics are sports data, pure and simple. Data is the fuel that ignites both excitement and disillusionment, pas-sion and indifference.

You need to realize that as much as this chapter is about a man's need to confront hard data, even the bare truth will not always convince him about oil usage. You have probably experienced this in your class presentations. You do a competent job delivering the information to those in attendance. No PowerPoint glitches. No fumbling for words. You masterfully touched on all your points and nailed your demonstrations like a convention speaker. You are prepared for all in attendance to eagerly swarm you to sign up, but instead, people politely say, "Thanks," and make a quick exit. You are mortified. What went wrong? You ask yourself, "How can sane people ignore this important information?" All that information poured out, and not one person is affected. While it does not seem possible, that scenario is only too common.

I have seen this phenomenon occur many times as a pastor of a church with regard to eternal issues. I would take great care to present the good news of Jesus to a gathering of people. I would explain very precisely how Jesus died on the cross to pay the penalty for the sins of all men. I would build a case detailing how Jesus rose from the grave and proved He is who He said He is—God. I would read from Bible verses like John 3:16, "For God so loved the world that He gave His only begotten Son, that whoever believes in Him will not perish but have everlasting life." I would tell them very plainly that when you believe He died in your place, God trades your sin for the righteousness of Jesus. That belief makes you forgiven of all sin, for all time, and you are granted eternal life as a free gift! You would think many a man (or woman) would jump at that offer. This information alone changed the culture of the entire western hemisphere! But sadly, many reject eternal life in spite of the facts. So you see, even with plenty of data backing up the health value of essential oils regarding physical life, many men still prefer to shrug it off and walk away unfazed.

So, what is it exactly that changes compiled facts and figures into something worth investing in? Faith! That's right—faith. Here is an example from the leisure realm: When a man comes to grips with all the data on his favorite sports team, it inspires his faith that they will improve, maybe even be very competitive in the coming season. With newfound faith anchored in all of this data, a sports fan might even believe his team can win a championship. This overdose of data makes the average fan into a super fan, willing to invest not only time in watching the team play but also in making an emotional investment. Hope springs eternal! With faith as a motivator, he buys T-shirts that proudly bear the name of his favorite team. He may purchase an oversized foam finger to wave wildly out of the car window while proclaiming his team to be number one. Due to the data, the fan has no shame! He defends the team's chances of winning against the challenges of others. He even endures the occasional mocking if his team loses badly.

The same can happen if a man's faith in essential oils can be inspired in connection to the data presented. With a little faith, he can transform the information you give him to not only use oils on occasion but even turn into a super oil fan. He may plunge into doing his own research. He can provide more knowledgeable support for your business. This super oil fan will one day be defending the cause and spitting out essential oil data to all comers!

This concept applies to a man's employment world as well. When data is compiled and organized, it becomes a resource that gives him the faith and confidence to go forward with a project, sale, or proposal. All the organized facts help create new products or improve and enhance old ones. The data might also warn of impending issues or outright failure, in which case a different course would need to be chosen altogether. In either case, a man is very comfortable making a decision once he has all the facts. Therefore, the more oil data you can find to answer his questions, the better your chances of motivating him to embrace oils.

Data mining is an essential piece of the puzzle that is securing the interest level of the average man. Keep this warning in mind, however—data is not gathered to win an argument but to encourage and inform! A man needs to feel respected, especially in the home. Giving him a verbal smack down with oil facts and making him feel inferior will not draw him closer to oil use. Dispense the information with humility and sensitivity for positive results. With a dump truck of data to plow through, he may just hit on something that grabs his attention, so don't be afraid to toss a few data points his way. Inspire his faith in essential oils by cunningly giving him plenty of supportive information at opportune times. You can throw out some interesting facts for him to mull over during dinner or while riding in the car. Encourage his belief that oils have the honest potential to help him feel more energetic, improve his sleep, and assist with chronic issues. Show him the stats!

History behind the oils is another great data source. Because the Bible contains many references to essential oils, their use can be traced back approximately six thousand years! Essential oils are hardly newcomers to the health and wellness scene. Do some research and find information that explains how and why past cultures used these oils. An Encyclopedia Britannica Online article from July 20, 1998, entitled *Essential Oil* states, "The first records of essential oils come from ancient India, Persia, and Egypt; and both Greece and Rome conducted extensive trade in odoriferous oils and ointments with the countries of the Orient." Depending upon how technical you want to be, or what you think your man will gravitate to, there are ample resources to provide data on the history and chemistry of oils. This would include data on the molecular structure of oils, oil compounds, elements that make up oils, and much more. For instance, does he know that the minute molecular structure of essential oils allows the oils to penetrate deeply into your system, penetrating even the blood-brain barrier, making the oils incredibly potent? Does he know oils are used worldwide, not just in your home and the homes of a few of your like-minded wacky friends? At the Young Living convention, some eye-opening data was shown. Does he know that there are millions of essential oil users and that over one hundred thousand joined last year alone? Have you given him examples of the many ways essential oils assist with soreness, stress, and pains and even serve in supporting emotional stability? Invest some energy in detailed research pin-pointing oils that will help his specific areas of need. He will respond faster to what works for him than to general information on what works. Do not attempt to be too cute; just lay some facts on him. If you want to be really subtle, accidentally on purpose leave some literature in the bathroom while removing other reading options. In time, he will become an oil scholar.

One area in the realm of interesting data connected to pure essential oils has to do with the benefits received when you use them. Another large aspect of data that is woefully underreported is what you do *not* get when you choose an oily lifestyle...negative side effects! My wife and I have been considering this important issue ever since I had cancer surgery twenty years ago. There are so many side effects with the myriad of drugs and treatments for cancer and surgery that I had to get relief from the cures! Like determined gold miners overcoming several setbacks, our continued searching and digging for toxin-free remedies and alternative health options led us to our essential oil discovery. We could not be more thrilled that not only can we use the oils in many various applications, but we also get the peace of mind that comes with the knowledge there are no harmful side effects connected with their appropriate use.

This is nowhere more apparent than when the two of us relax for the night in front of some classic old movie. We witness the many commercials touting breakthrough pharmaceutical products that have thirty seconds of product advertising and two minutes of side-effect disclaimers. We cannot help but laugh out loud when we see an advertisement for an antidepressant medication with side effects, including, "May cause suicidal tendencies." Say *what*? For one arthritis medication, the side effects were so numerous I could not believe it. So, I did what all inquiring people do when they have a question: I Googled it! I found my answer on Drugs.com. In my wildest dreams, I could not have imagined that the side effects of this product were actually a longer list on paper than the already outrageous list they recited in the television version. It took *seven pages* to print out the side effect information of the one drug. The information was broken down into four particular lists, including the more common major side effects of which eighteen were listed. Then came the less common major side effects of which ninety-six were listed—yes, that's *ninety-six*! As if to make the consumer feel better about actually ingesting the medication, the minor side effects were then listed, including twenty more common ones and nineteen less common ones. Whew! That is a whopping total of 153 possible side effects connected with just one pharmaceutical medication. The amazing thing is the ridiculous portrayal of happy, smiling people as the disclaimer of tragic side effects is recited. Can you really be smiling if you are suffering from body aches and pains, stomach pain, lightheadedness, nasal congestion, pain or tenderness around the eyes or cheekbones, shivering, trouble sleeping, and rapid and sometimes shallow breathing added to the original arthritic condition you suffer from? In addition to this are the exponential risks associated with taking drugs in combination. How long do they think people will be duped by this foolishness?

The following sad tale illustrates the side effect risks of multiplied drugs. Not long ago my aging uncle was suffering due to changes in his blood pressure medication. The doctors then assigned him an additional medication to counter the original medication. This combination of drugs left him lethargic and tired. He was active and still employed into his late eighties, but this situation forced him into retirement. More medication was prescribed, and soon his appetite was all but gone. All of this sent him into a bit of depression, for which additional medication was given. No joke! Constant tiredness, loss of appetite, and depression were not conducive to long life. Thankfully, after seeking a second opinion from a more thorough doctor, all the medications were removed, and his original blood pressure medication was tweaked, and *shazam!* He is like a new man. Without all the unnecessary medications and multiplied side effects, he has resumed travel, gardening, and is enjoying life. He is no longer resigned to a life of sluggishness and gloom. He is now applying multiple oils as needed and has restored energy and vibrancy into his daily routine.

Contrast the aforementioned information of multiplied side effects associated with drug usage with the side effects connected with essential oil usage. The short answer is that there are no harmful side effects with pure essential oils! Derived from the natural components in plants, essential oils work with our bodies, not against them. Hooray! When an authentic, therapeutic grade essential oil is placed on the skin or inhaled, there are no harmful side effects. Even when oils are used in combination we find that they are safe. As stated by Dr. David Stewart in his book, *The Chemistry of Essential Oils Made Simple*, "Hazardous interactions between different essential oils applied together are unheard of."

Any reference to side effects with regard to essential oils seems to be from testing done on fragrance-grade oils and less-than-pure samples. Even when an allergic reaction to an oil is reported, it can often be traced back to the low grade of the oil and the impurities contained in it. The proper use and dosage of pure, therapeutic-grade essential oils can enhance all the systems of your body without producing hazardous side effects!

This is where Young Living's Seed to Seal process pays big dividends. In the whole scheme of things, this is important data for men to know. As the purity of the oil is a key to its effectiveness, no one else in the industry can claim as high a standard due, in part, to Young Living owning its own farms. Young Living cares for the soil without chemical fertilizers and grows the plants without applying harmful pesticides. Crops are harvested at the most favorable time, and plants are distilled at the optimum moment when the plant will release the most oils. Now, that is some solid data for men to breathe in! Young Living tests and retests throughout the process and then tests for impurities again after bottling. Whew! If some men are still in doubt, plan a road trip to one of the farms so he can collect his own facts. All that to say, when you pick up a bottle of Peppermint oil, you can be certain it is pure, therapeutic-grade Peppermint. That's the kind of data that will make a man want to grab a bottle! There is a commercial where a certain fast-food chain claims, "We have the meats." Well, because of the Seed to Seal purity process, Young Living can proclaim, "We have the farms!" Time for a mic drop!

Obviously there is a mountain of data to sort through related to essential oils. Men need proper data to make a proper decision. You can find significant data, no matter the angle you are researching from or the interest level of the one you are providing it for. Remember, don't use the data simply to triumph in an argument but rather to patiently and masterfully influence and inform.

THE LAST DROP

Ladies, this is a critical piece to a man's essential oil journey with you. Do not smother him with data, but be prepared to answer honest questions. Choose choice morsels of data that might truly speak to your husband's needs or interests and creatively enlighten him. The light will come on eventually!

Okay, men, here is your turn to be challenged. Take a deep breath and educate yourself about essential oils, Young Living, and current health and wellness issues. Do not categorically dismiss oils without any knowledge on the subject. Do not minimize information that comes from your wife. She is the one learning. You need to catch up.

"I married Mrs. Right. I just didn't know
her first name was Always!"

—Anonymous

"Life is too short to remove USB safely."

—Anonymous

"If you start now, you'll see results one day
earlier than if you wait until tomorrow."

—Anonymous

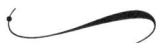

Chapter 6

Desperate Times...
Desperate Measures

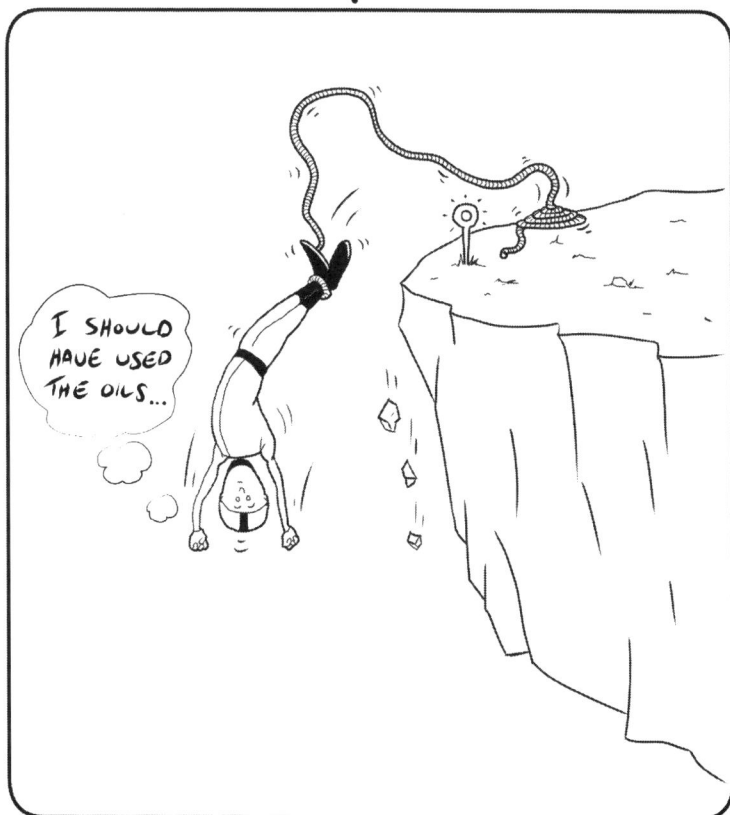

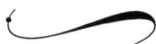

"And they were casting out many demons
and were anointing with oil many sick
people and healing them."

—MARK 6:13

"Is anyone among you sick? Let him call
for the elders of the church, and let them
pray over him, anointing him with oil in
the name of the Lord..."

—JAMES 5:14

"Dost thou love life? Then do not squander
time for that is the stuff life is made of."

—BENJAMIN FRANKLIN

"Only a fool would underestimate a man
with nothing to lose."

—LANCE CONRAD

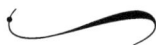

6

DESPERATE TIMES...DESPERATE MEASURES

THE MOST SUCCESSFUL way for a man to acquiesce to applying essential oils seems to be during a time of dire, back-against-the-wall, no-other-option crisis! Catch him at a weak moment, like when sick or hurt and willing to try anything for relief of his discomfort. It is never easy for a man to admit a wrong or a mis-calculation. Resist trying to convince him he is wrong. Wait for that golden opportunity when he needs your help to make it through the most severe tummy ache anyone ever had or the nasal congestion even Hannibal the Great couldn't conquer. Trust me, that moment will come! A man is a peculiar character. He can in one moment be the most macho, awe-inspiring, energetic, athletic soldier and statesman you ever laid eyes on. The very same man with a common cold or an upset stomach reverts to Mamma's little boy who needs lots of TLC in a big hurry. I may or may not be speaking from experience.

In chapter 1 I mentioned my introduction to oils story that my wife shared in a class context. Let me share my story with you, as it applies to this chapter's discussion. I was one of those skeptical guys who was not interested in hearing about essential oils and was even less interested in their use. Diane did not corner me into using them, and we never argued about it. I would mostly just avoid the subject, and she would look for opportunities to gently provide info and sample drops or sniffs. She had received her Premium Starter Kit and was being educated voraciously on all things oils and their particular uses for health purposes. Over the ten months she had been using oils, she had tried to get me to use them, but she did not push them on me. I barely paid any attention to the oils. She raved about how Peppermint had played a role in reducing her migraine issues and that she loved how other oils helped support a better night's sleep. Diane was reading oil reference books and constantly watching many videos online. I was oblivious. I didn't know anything about the oils and was satisfied in my ignorance. So I thought.

I had cancer surgery twenty years ago to remove an abdominal tumor. Ever since that surgery, I have had digestive issues from post-op intestinal paralysis. My physician instructed me to give it time, and things would go back to normal, but no matter how long I waited, normalcy never returned. I waited eighteen years. Since that time, we searched for ways to regulate my system along with eating better and living healthier. At times I would have success, but it was temporary at best. The hard-to-predict extremes of my digestion were worrisome to manage. I made several trips to the hospital over the years to get my stomach pumped when things got too stopped up. Like a line from an old TV show, this was literally "up my nose with a rubber hose." I do not recommend this tortuous procedure to anyone! Forget conventional forms of torturing the enemy. This is the method the military should use to get prisoners to "talk." I think stomach pumping was invented at the same time as the rack and thumb screws.

In the fall of 2015, I was feeling my stomach tightening up, and dread set upon me as I assumed I would need to return to the hospital to get my stomach pumped again. Whatever products I had used to head off the problem were not working. My wife knew I was hurting, because I came home from work at mid-day, which I never do. Plopping down in a chair at the kitchen table, I was so disappointed to concede I would need to go back to the hospital for another hose job. She was feeling my pain. I was feeling my pain even more. In that moment she got a twinkle in her eye as she remembered her essential oils. This time she confidently told me there was a specific oil called Digize that she had in her kit that could help relieve my stomach issues. I was too despondent to argue and in too much pain to care, so I agreed to try some. She applied a few drops of Digize and Peppermint (also a good digestive oil and magnifier of other oils) to my abdomen. Of all the oils to begin with, Digize did not have a very appealing scent. I was not very confident of any positive outcome, but I was desperate!

The good news is that despite my hesitancy, once the oils were applied, I began to have abdominal noises within 10 minutes, which sounded like music to my ears. Something was happening after all. In a little while we added another dose, figuring we might get even more results. Sure enough, an hour later I was back to work. Indeed, desperate times called for des-perate measures, but that application of oils made a believer out of me without ever having to argue about it. I have not been back to the hospital since. The benefit of the oils helping to balance my system also means I do not have to apply them often to keep my system under control. My wife did not gloat or in any way give me the "I told you so" speech; however, I was totally happy that she did rub it in. Pun intended!

Over the last couple of years, I have been learning to incorporate many essential oils and oil-infused products into my routine. Lemon drops in my water to start the day. Breathe Again blend to assist my air intake when I go running. Cool Azul or Deep Relief to help soothe my aches and pains from work or sports. Digize to keep my digestion in check. Stress Away to support good night's sleep. I also love Thieves! I'm not talking about the people who take multiple samples but never actually sign up. I'm referring to the oil blend. I use Thieves for added support in many health applications. And then there's Idaho Blue Spruce to help support testosterone production for, you know... running. And it all started when I became desperate enough to let a drop of oil touch me!

I do not consider myself an exception in this case. I believe many men will keep the oils at arm's length, or farther, until they really need help, and then desperation will motivate them to give them a try. You may take the opportunity to suggest a six-week, eight-week, or three-month protocol for him to try. During this time, he can collect his own data on the results he gets. Once he sees positive results, his skepticism will diminish. I have heard varying accounts from other men—maybe not to the same extreme, but many of them had waited to try the oils until they had no other options. Let me share with you a few of these revealing stories. The following are responses I received on an oils-for-dudes Facebook page after I asked for men's introductory oil experiences.

Aaron from California wrote; "My original 'sold moments' were all on the immediate product benefits: Immupro for sleep, Digize for nausea and Peppermint for fever." He also added an emergency-for-dad tale. Evidently, his seven-year-old and two-year-old boys were in the same room and playing instead of going to sleep. (That hardly ever happens!) He continued to say that he gave each of them one-fourth of an Immupro tablet and began reading them a story. They were out in fifteen minutes! When products rescue Dad and help the children, it is a double win. On a side note, Aaron was also pleasantly surprised at the extra pick-me-up that a drop of Peppermint in his morning coffee provided.

In a couple more similar desperation cases, another responder to my Facebook question said he was

YOU CAN LEAD A MAN TO OILS...

hunched over and in "immense pain" in his lower back because of a degenerative condition. His wife applied some Peppermint to the painful area. He was then able to straighten up! Since then, he has not looked back. The next responder said he had a cold and wanted a sinus rinse. His wife put a drop of both RC and Peppermint in the rinse, and he was sold! The significance of that "sale" is that this man is a pharmacist, and he comes from a "LONG line of pharmacists" who own their own businesses. He knows that medicines were at one time plant-based, so it was not a difficult transition. Another remarkable story he shared was the "TONS" of change they have witnessed with their son who has ADD. It seems the oils have helped to support what he calls "stellar" focus. When guys see relief for their children, it is clearly a motivator to start using oils.

Some guys are still unwilling to give them a try or to pay much attention to the oil thing happening with their wives. But their day of enlightenment will come. When that day of desperation comes, ladies, have your oils at the ready and let it drop! Aside from the lost time of using the oils because of various, made-up excuses, the good thing about this scenario is that once a man receives the benefits of using the essential oils, he's in for life. In my case, no one can take that experience away or convince me to turn from oil usage with negative info, because I know they work. These men know it too.

There is another daring desperate measure for you to employ. There is an old adage in sales that women would do well to heed, especially if their man stubbornly resists discussing or using essential oils. That age-old, genius approach to sales and marketing is simply this: sex sells! This is not rocket science, and neither is it new news. Television, movies, magazines, and many other types of sales and marketing campaigns successfully employ the sex angle on a daily basis. Why wouldn't women who are encouraging husbands to try essential oils benefit from it as well? So, ladies, no matter how hopeless your man seems or how oblivious he has remained to all the oil products, their uses, and the hype, you still have your greatest tool in the proverbial toolbox. The power of sex is a power like no other.

Let me make a cautionary statement here for clarification purposes. I am in no way suggesting that a woman use sex in any form or fashion as a punishment to her husband until or unless he succumbs to oil usage. That tactic is off limits! Trust me when I say that any move in that direction could be detrimental to your marriage. Hurt feelings, resentment, and misunderstanding could send the whole discussion spiraling in a direction that was never intended. Therefore, be very careful how you play with this fire. A burn in this area of your marriage can leave lasting scars.

That being understood, there are some advantages a woman has to get her man, let's say, highly interested in essential oils. It may also be fair and downright honest to say that he can most definitely be stimulated to give the oils more serious consideration. Ladies, I have warned in a previous chapter that sticking a bottle of oil in your man's face to have him smell the oil and react to the fragrance is not a beneficial or productive tactic. However, placing some of the oils on yourself at the proper time, in the proper place, can make for sudden interest in and attraction to oils. "I don't want you smelling good and stirring my passions while we're in bed," said no man ever! He doesn't even have to know at first that it is the oils that he is enjoying. You can enlighten him once he inquires about that particular fragrance he has noticed or has asked for you to use again. You can even let him put the oils on you, which can be very provocative. He will subtly learn that touching the oils will not bring on the apocalypse. Since association plays a big part in acceptance, his association of oil fragrances with your times of intimacy will dramatically alter his attention to the matter and make it a pleasing topic to ponder. As men think about sex a great deal, you will have found a way to your man's heart even faster than through his stomach. Bow-chick-a-bow-wow! Yes, there are oils for everything.

And what man in his right mind (if that's not an oxymoron) would refuse a massage after a hard day's work? He may not ask, but you can occasionally offer. Men like to know that their hard work is appreciated, and offering a rubdown can set a good tone. He may vacate at the first sign of an oil conversation, but he will not move when you start massaging. At moments like these, he is vulnerable to embrace the power of the drop! Certainly this would be a perfect time to place a few drops of oil on your hands and rub them on in a gentle, soothing fashion. Yeah, I'm thinking that he will not only enjoy that, but he may also start dropping hints that he wants you to do that again…soon. Like a fly caught in a spider's web, you've got him!

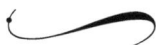

THE LAST DROP
Ladies, this may in fact be where the proverbial rubber "meets the road." His desperation may be the best time to introduce essential oils and let him experience their impact. Remember that you can also create an intimate desperation for him. All is fair in love and oils!

Gentlemen, most of you will experience some form of desperation. Don't resist the opportunity to see first-hand what the oils can do. Oils support health and a whole lot more. You have heard how they have worked for others. Now it is your turn to move out of essential oil darkness and into the light.

"If you don't design your own life's plan, chances are you'll fall into someone else's plan. And guess what they have planned for you? Not much!"

—JIM ROHN

"Behold the turtle, he makes progress only when he sticks his neck out."

—ANONYMOUS

"Knowledge is knowing a tomato is a fruit. Wisdom is not putting it in a fruit salad."

—ANONYMOUS

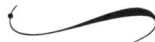

Chapter 7

Minding Her Own Business

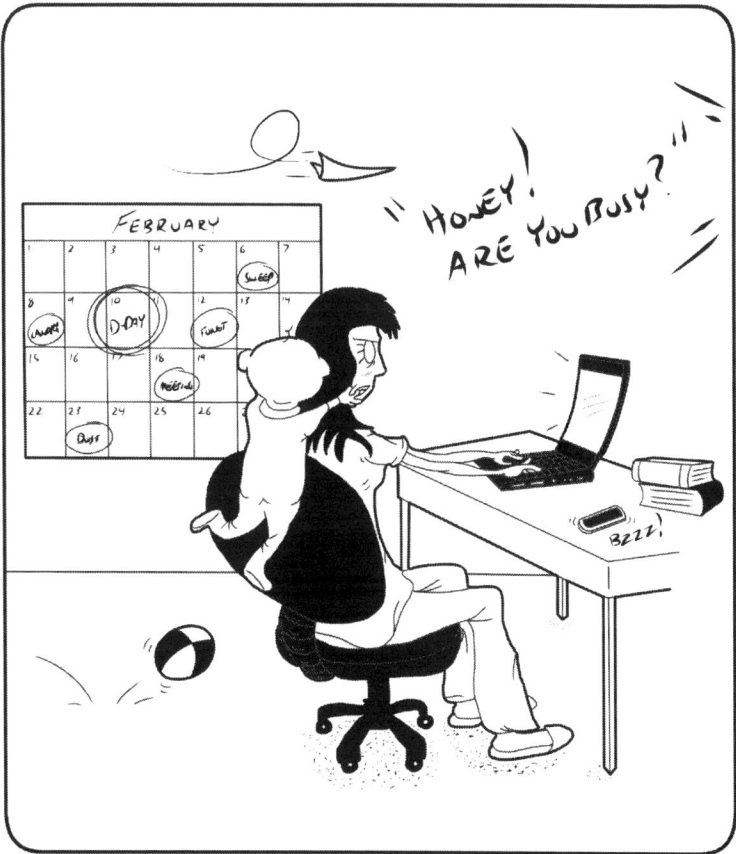

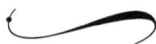

"An excellent wife, who can find? For her worth is far above jewels.

The heart of her husband trusts in her, And he will have no lack of gain...

She rises also while it is still night, And gives food to her household, And portions to her maidens.

She considers a field and buys it; From her earnings she plants a vineyard...

Strength and dignity are her clothing, And she smiles at the future...

She looks well to the ways of her household, And does not eat the bread of idleness."

—PROVERBS *31:10–27*

"One reason we are so harried and hurried is that we make yesterday and tomorrow our business, when all that legitimately concerns us is today."

—ELISABETH ELIOT

"...The best thing we can do is start a home-based business."

—DAVE RAMSEY

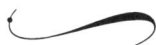

7

MINDING HER OWN BUSINESS

IF A PICTURE is worth a thousand words, then take another close look at the picture illustrating this chapter. That picture speaks volumes about what the average woman who begins an essential oil business handles on a daily basis. It may, in fact, be understated. The business side of essential oil use has been touched on a few times in other chapters, but I have not given it proper attention...until now. I have seen firsthand the effort and dedication being poured out to start and keep the business going. Unfortunately, many husbands are oblivious to the business venture and all its responsibilities that are going on in the same house. I'll say more on this a bit later. For you ladies who are undertaking a Young Living oil business, I applaud you. The props you deserve are probably long overdue. For you guys who have wives building a business, there is a lot going on. You really need to pay more attention!

Let's begin with the idea of effort. A large number of women who begin this oil network marketing business may already have a full-time job or two. Young, working moms are doing quite the balancing act. There are household needs, which may include tending to little ones, preparing meals, and keeping the house tidy. If it's anything like my house, there is always laundry to be done. Work outside the home has its own requirements. When there is finally a restful moment, these energetic moms take on their own oil business assignments. On some days the whirlwind of activity is so intense that desks are left cluttered, sinks are filled with dirty dishes, phone calls are left unanswered, and the script for the next presentation is staring you in the face...unfinished. At times, not even Pinterest can provide the solution. But amazingly, in the nick of time, the priority items get accomplished. No guilt should be attached to any residual things that are left undone. Any of these roles is enough responsibility for one person, but when all three are being performed at the same time, that is nothing short of Wonder Woman material!

There are other women who begin a business when their children are grown or already out of the home. Once again, they are to be commended for taking on this new business challenge instead of resting in their empty nests. Phone calls, meeting preparations, education, strategy sessions, presentations, team support—all add up to maximum effort being infused into the business. This is not an easy step to take, but they jumped in with both feet. Well done, ladies!

For some of you, the business actually happens unexpectedly. When you became a Young Living member, you had no intention of selling the products or starting a business. You were just excited to use the products themselves and build on the education you were acquiring. But with results came sharing the news with others. You knew plenty of people who would also benefit from essential oil usage, so you started sharing with those you care about. Seeing the needs of others and meeting them is a large part of the oil lifestyle that excites people. Squeee! What fun! Before you knew it, checks began to arrive in the mail. You got an adrenaline boost, because getting checks is always more fun than writing them. At some point you had to make the decision to make it a business. Suddenly, you are off and running.

Many of you have taken a more direct approach to this network marketing opportunity. Upon hearing about the business and seeing the results in the lives of other oil users, you knew right away you would make a go of the business. Good for you! It's great when a plan comes together. In either case, whether you slid into the business slowly or you dove in right away, it is understood that there is a lot of effort being put out. Keep up the good work!

No one starts a network marketing business just for the love of effort. You have a significant reason that you began your essential oil business—it has definite income potential. (There I go again, blurting out the truth!) This is a point not to be ignored. Although it is sometimes awkward to talk about publicly, writing about it is quite easy. And while downplaying the income your business produces may be prudent, it is a fact that we all need money, and we diligently work in some fashion to get it. You can take comfort in knowing your dedicated effort will be rewarded with a satisfying payday. No matter how much or how little emphasis you wish to place on the income, George Bailey (*It's a Wonderful Life*) said it best when he reminded the angel, "It comes in pretty handy down here, Bub!"

It is worth noting that many women sign up for a
Premium Starter Kit and never intend to sell essential oils or have a business. As a matter of fact, they
never do! According to Young Living's 2016 Income
Disclosure Statement (IDS), 94 percent of members
stay at the distributor level. Getting discounts on
the products has its own value, to be sure, so there
is nothing wrong with that decision. This does show,
however, that if you have taken on an oil business, you
are among the 6 percent who have decided to tackle
the extra challenge.

For the women in the 6 percent business group, the
sky is the limit as far as income potential. According to
the IDS, the range of yearly income starts at just above
nine hundred dollars and peaks at almost two million! I think I can find something to put that money
toward. You probably can too. Most likely, there are
a number of guys reading this who just picked their
jaws up from the floor. Yes, the earnings potential is
that enormous! This is why your wife would enjoy your
support. Now here's some news for you. You won't
reach that level in a week or a month, and probably
not in a year. But the good news is that you can attain
it. The key word is "potential." The money is out there
to be made, and it all boils down to what you make of
the opportunity. In this direct selling format, there

is really nothing holding you back. So aim high and don't give up!

When you dove into your essential oil business, you were encouraged to have a "Why." Any four-year-old will ask you "Why?" one hundred times a day. Although he or she may not realize it at the time, it is a very powerful question. Your personal "why" is the reason you decided to start this business. This will not only serve as the goal you're ultimately aiming for, but it also becomes your motivation along the way. Remember that there are as many "whys" as there are women doing the business. All "whys" are personal and matter greatly. Stay focused on your "why"; don't get sidetracked by someone else's. Some women start with a simple "why" to earn enough money to pay for their own oils. That is a super agenda and, when that goal is realized, can be very satisfying. Other "whys" are more complex and may take years to accomplish. Some ladies want to become debt free, bless others monetarily, or donate to specific ministries. Others have goals for college funds for their children or grandchildren. There are ladies who are aiming at extra money for travel or other leisure activities. All of these are worthy goals, indeed.

"Whys" can also fluctuate, especially when your initial "why" comes to fruition. This is expected as life furnishes changes along your business venture. Embrace the changes and enjoy the journey. Whether you're in business to pay for your oils, retire some debt, or retire your husband, I encourage you to share your "why" with your husband often. In this way, he can be catching the vision along with you. And it just might soften his stance on essential oils, knowing you've designed your efforts to help him.

Another prominent feature of building your essential oil business is the built-in self-improvement package. Yes, having your own business stretches you in ways you never imagined. Let's face it. For most people, you fill out an application and find a job that "fits" you. The job is in an area you're already comfortable with, and you are not regularly asked to perform duties outside of your comfort zone. You clock in and clock out without dramatic changes in a zombie-like routine. The boss does not push you to grow, and coworkers are happy when things don't change. It is a safe place, and the challenges are limited. Well, having your own business is nothing quite as conventional as all that. I'm going to go out on a limb here and say that many of you have found out that a large amount of personal growth has already come your way since you started your business.

Several areas are responsible for bringing about that growth. The first is all the different people you meet with varied needs, interests, and motivations. Your little world opens up in a hurry. The stereotypes you once had get dashed to pieces, and a new learning curve is created. It is fascinating to see how different people talk, work, practice their faith, dream, and get motivation. You've heard that you should "never judge a book by its cover," but now, more than ever, you can see the significance of that phrase. People you least expected have shown the most amazing talents. Shy people blossom, and the loud ones turn out to be soft as marshmallows and they show great compassion. You learn so much without even trying.

Education is a second factor that moves you to personal growth. Depending on the individual and how deep of a researcher you are, there are so many opportunities to learn and grow. Guys, I'm being straight up with you when I say you should be impressed with all the knowledge your wife has acquired. She's a walking oil library! She has discovered and most likely read numerous books on the kinds of oils, the chemistry of oils, and the assorted sciences behind essential oils working in unity with your bodily chemistry. Some women actually enjoy that chemistry kind of stuff!

There are books about oils and pets. There are books about oils and children. There are also educational videos to help you in your presentations, classes, suggested oil usage, and all sorts of DIY hacks. You get the idea. It seems the more you learn, the more you want to learn. Getting a starter kit should come with a degree for all the learning that takes place. Can I get an "Amen!"?

I don't want to sugarcoat this too much. Clearly your business is not all fun and learning. So let me talk for a moment about the challenges you face with your business. Time is always a factor, and being organized enough to learn, prepare, plan, and then present a class can be very challenging for most—especially at first, when all of this is new and resources are scarce. The time crunch factor never really goes away. The planned schedule gets bumped by the tyranny of the urgent, and it is difficult to get things reeled in again. It is helpful that Young Living is now making website capabilities available for their distributors. There is also a third-party web builder available that lets you compose your own personal website. You can see an illustration of this website, what it provides, and gain exposure to many educational videos by logging onto www.yldist.com/oilsymphony. Anything that helps simplify your life is a blessing.

The next challenge is the emotional crisis of overcoming your own sense of inadequacy. You know the drill—comparing your presentation with someone else's and feeling yours was inferior. Or you're watching someone else's video and feeling paralyzed by fear to put one out there yourself. You have braced yourself through the criticism of non-oil users. You continued on toward your goals in spite of doubters. You have learned to carry lots of stuff without help. Yes, you deserve to be commended for overcoming those challenges and moving forward. You have had to hurdle additional obstacles like scheduling, marketing, strategizing, and team building. Maybe some of you don't even realize all the ways you've been stretched since you began your business, but believe me, it is noticeable, and you're all the better for it. There are so many men asking, "What happened to my quiet, reserved wife? Watching her come out of her shell is amazing!" You should feel energized about all your growth too.

All of your personal growth is amazing and part of the rewards that come with your own essential oil business. Yes, I said "rewards." Maybe you need a quick summary of your rewards about now to strengthen and encourage you. The personal growth you've experienced is a huge reward. You will have new coping skills and life lessons to lean on in the future. The growing income is a reward that you have earned. Enjoy that reward! There is no guilt connected to what you earn due to your investment of hard work.

One of the biggest rewards, and one that you may appreciate more as time goes on, is the friendships that are forged through your business venture. You've met like-minded people who are passionate about the same things. They understand and accept you. That is a reward like no other! And, unfortunately, lost in all the day-to-day hustle and bustle and business scurrying is the starting point of the entire oil journey. A most remarkable reward is the joy and increased wellness that has come to your household and to many others through your efforts. High fives all around!

All the rewards mentioned previously should make you men realize that your lack of endorsement hurts you and your wife in several ways. When you stubbornly hold out against the use of essential oils, you're keeping yourself at arm's length from a lot of wonderful people who are also associated with essential oils. You may even be guilty of unintentionally holding back your support for your wife's business. You may be giving her shallow emotional support when what she needs is some big-time help to overcome doubts or fears. You're making her mind her own business when you could be assisting. She could probably benefit from some of your expertise that would help her business thrive. Don't wait until you're sleeping on the couch to figure out she needs your help! Willingly giving your physical, emotional, and spiritual support would be a rich reward to her. She desires to grow the business with you, not in spite of you.

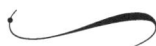

THE LAST DROP

Ladies, don't ever feel second rate or consider giving up on your business. Just the fact that you took the leap into your own business speaks volumes about your strength and determination. Stay determined to meet the challenges as they come, but take time to enjoy the rewards too.

Guys, here's the deal. This business is so important to your wife for many reasons—reasons like her self-esteem, her desires for the future, and her wellness now, just to name a few. Don't let her down. Make a conscious decision to be of whatever help you can and watch her business soar.

"*When my kids become wild and unruly, I use a nice, safe playpen. When they're finished, I climb out.*"

—ERMA BOMBECK

"*Money can't buy happiness, but it sure makes misery easier to live with.*"

—ANONYMOUS

"*Money talks...but all mine ever says is 'good bye.'*"

—ANONYMOUS

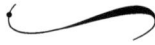

Chapter 8

C'Mon, Man!

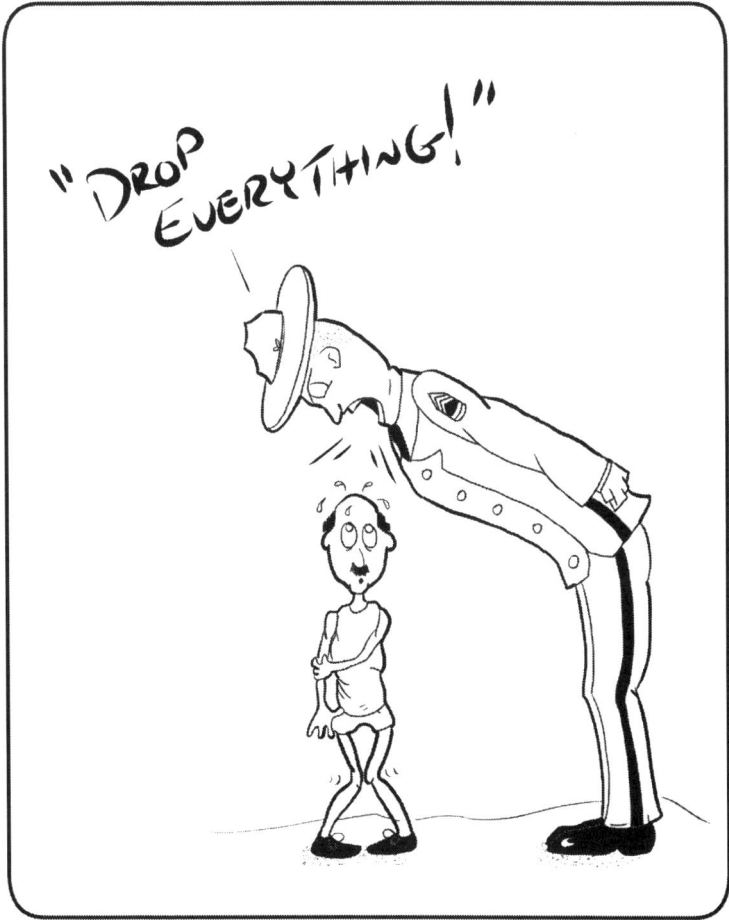

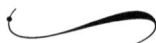

"Be on the alert, stand firm in the faith, act like men, be strong."

—1 CORINTHIANS 16:13

"Truth makes many appeals, not the least of which is the power to shock."

—JULES RENARD, FRENCH WRITER

"Procrastination is like a credit card, it's a lot of fun until you get the bill."

—CHRISTOPHER PARKER

"Necessity is the mother of taking chances."

—MARK TWAIN

8

C'MON, MAN!

UP UNTIL NOW, I've done a lot of kidding around about the subject and maybe, to some degree, given men a legit rationale, or maybe an excuse, for their resistance. That, my male friends, is not my intent. Rather than give you a way out, I am trying to push you in! The lighthearted approach was aimed at getting you to laugh at the situation as it is. All the while, I've tried to convince you it is quite a bit of foolishness to ignore sound advice and forego healthy living. To be frank, this is no laughing matter. To say your health is important may be the understatement of a lifetime. Think about it. Your health affects every aspect of your life. Your health is important to your wife, your children, your employer, your extended family, and your friends. If you are approximately my age, maybe your health is important to your grandchildren too.

Men can find a myriad of ways to distract themselves. Whether it is by something as benign as falling asleep in front of the TV, watching sports for hours, or participating in an active hobby or athletic activity, men tend to keep busy. Some men are grease monkeys and keep themselves busy in the garage. Many these days are computer geeks and can be found tinkering with the hard drive or adding another gadget to an already crowded array. Some men run, fish, hunt, climb, and so on. Like busy minions, men mean well with their activities but may not be accomplishing anything of real value. None of these activities is bad, and actually, many are quite good. However, it is imperative for men to make a distinction between the "good" things in life and the "valuable" things. To emphasize the good over the valuable is a huge mistake. The valuable things that you need to give priority to in your life include spiritual depth, your own health and well-being, and certainly the wellness of your family. I hate to break it to you, but Netflix is *not* a valuable thing. What *is* invaluable is to understand your wife and find ways to fortify and reassure her. There is no phone app you can download to do this for you. You must invest brain power and emotional energy the old-fashioned way. Her use of essential oils should be important to you, if only because it is important to her. Though it may be hard to concede time away from your normal distractions, you will soon reap the benefits of this mind-set.

Take another look at the Bible verse that was quoted at the beginning of this chapter. One of the marvels of Scripture is that not only is there spiritual value in what is written, but there is physical value as well. So let's take real-life applications from these words.

*Be on the alert. Don't duck out on your responsibility to stay alert. The verse was written for us to be alert to spiritual pitfalls, but there are plenty of other dangers you need to be alert to. For instance, your wife needs to be loved. Be alert to make sure she is getting plenty of it...from you. Never let anything, including oil issues, deprive her of your love. Regarding a healthy lifestyle, are you aware of the many toxins and chemicals in the food you regularly purchase and consume? Fertilizers, insect sprays, dyes, and so much more are included in the American diet. Processing of the foods takes out most, if not all, of the nutritional value, and then vitamins are artificially reintroduced. Have you spent any time considering pharmaceuticals? Are you alert to the dangerous side effects of drugs, vaccines, and medications being prescribed these days? It is not just your wife's job to protect the family but yours as well.

*Stand firm in the faith. Originally, this was an admonition to bear up under pressure when Christian beliefs were challenged. But again, a physical application would be instructive here. There are a multitude of skeptics regarding essential oils and network marketing. Your wife will unfairly face ridicule, judgment, and possibly poor treatment for her involvement with essential oils. Will you stand with her and support her through it all? She needs you. This quote by Billy Graham says it well: "Courage is contagious. When a brave man takes a stand, the spines of others are often stiffened." Educate yourself on Young Living's Seed to Seal quality assurance. You will be amazed at the lengths they go through to ensure they are putting out the purest oil in the industry! Oils work. Check out the many personal testimonies that will help reinforce why these are called *essential* oils. Your wife needs you to stand with her.

*Act like men. When that was written two thousand years ago, I'm sure there was a certain picture the readers would get in their minds as to what good qualities the average man should possess. Here are a few to consider: The first would be integrity. Integrity is doing the right thing even when no one is looking. So make a concentrated effort to aim at wellness, even if no one else approves or understands. The next is boldness. Meeting challenges head on is expected of a man. Life is not a simple journey. In no area of life do people get a free pass to easy living. Stuff happens. Acting like a man means having the boldness to speak the truth in love, adapting to change, and supporting others, particularly your family, through the hardships. Using essential oils and adapting to a new, healthy lifestyle may be strange and intimidating but, guys, act like men!

Although there are many other traits that I could list, the final one I will discuss is honesty. To act like a man is to be honest. Honestly evaluate your current lifestyle. Is it working? Are you healthy, or are you in steady decline? Would you like to improve your health? Would you like to improve your financial situation (see appendix for Income Disclosure Statement)? Being resigned to your lifestyle or conditioned to it is not honesty; it is surrender at best and neglect at worst. Don't give up when hope is available. Don't give in when instead you can overcome. Experience what the power of a drop can do!

*Be strong. Our culture seems to be sissifying males wherever and whenever possible. This is your opportunity to resist that trend. I beg you, cease purchasing man rompers! Level one for a man involved with essential oils is to carry things! Your wife is loading the car for classes, setting up vendor booths, and receiving large boxes in the mail. Be strong for her. Carry stuff!

A second area of strength is found in the truth that living healthy, exercising, eating right, and using essential oils is not wimpy, unmanly, or in any way soft. Sometimes, being strong is not merely a display of brute force but a compilation of wise actions, steady character, and the resolve to do what is right. You can be that man!

Another way to be strong for your woman is to help ward off naysayers and complainers. Be her best cheerleader. Convince your wife to believe she is a Royal Crown Diamond, no matter what her rank. Strengthen her resolve to move forward through discouraging times. Be strong by having your own testimony of how the oils have helped you. No one can take away or depreciate your story! Be strong by educating yourself on healthy living. Replace toxins with healthy alternatives. Visit the Young Living farms and learn how their process protects the products. Attend the next convention with your wife. You will encourage her and at the same time be overwhelmed with a new appreciation for all that essential oils and the Young Living Corporation are accomplishing in people's lives. Research the uses and results of essential oils and build your resolve so you can be strong no matter what criticism comes your way. Your woman will draw from that strength and love you for it!

With that being said, men, you need to come down from the ledge and "man up" to essential oils. Think about all the rough-and-tumble activities you have been involved in. Over the years, you have participated in sports activities from soccer to football, baseball, fishing, camping, hunting, and hiking. Maybe even the work you do has its share of risks, injuries, and smelly slop that gets on you or on your clothes. With any of these, you've gotten your share of bumps, bruises, and breaks that you've worn like a badge of honor. Yet somehow, rubbing a drop of oil on your skin seems so terrifying! Really? You've probably endured painful or uncomfortable remedies in the past, like shots, sprays, and pills to gag on. You were brave enough for those. What happened?

Now think with me about the many other substances you rub on or apply to yourself without thought of consequences. For instance, many of you still apply shaving cream to your faces. Some of you rub gels or mousse in your hair. Depending upon where you live, some may have the opportunity to regularly apply sunscreen. And there are always the bug repellents or deodorant sprays you frequently apply. Some of you may be hunters and apply gross, unmentionable liquids to make you smell like the animal you are hunting. There are many, I'm sure, who have gone through the interesting, if not painful, tattooing process. Most of you have not even considered how toxic these things may be to your body, but on it goes. Now you're asked to rub on a drop or two of essential oil, and you put up all kinds of barriers or make all kinds of arguments to justify your ignorance. C'mon, man, you don't really know why you don't want to try oils—you just naturally resist. Stop it! Quit making lame excuses and use the oils. Do the right thing, and risk the consequences!

Another aspect to consider in this day and age is health-care insurance. Many today are finding that their health-care insurance provided through their employer is actually providing less and costing more. (Don't get me started!) Some are losing health insurance altogether or finding it difficult to get help when needed. Due to the current upheaval in health care, many insurance companies and employers are

incentivizing preventative health and wellness measures. Some reward those who work out regularly.
Others encourage their employees to wear tracking
devices to measure their daily steps or lose weight
and encourage a less sedentary lifestyle. (Yes, that's
what those devices are for, not so your employer can
track the length of your lunch break.) Employers are
providing healthy lunch and snack choices, and some
are providing in-house gyms. Here is another area
wherein essential oils can play a mighty role—preventative health care. Incorporating these oils in your
daily routine can help support a better physical condition. There are essential oils and oil-infused supplements that support every system in your body. By
experiencing less health complications, the need for
expensive health care can be reduced. Instead of an
apple a day, you should strongly consider some oils a
day. Who knows—with the wave of essential oil users
ever increasing, employers and insurance companies
may even start subsidizing their use!

In the past centuries, it was kings, priests, and wise
men who possessed the oils and dispensed them. Oils
were valued for health purposes and fragrant aromas.
Because of that value, oils were often used as a type
of currency. These influential men knew that the oils'
value was in their natural potency to work with our

bodily systems, not against them. Over the centuries, men have abdicated that knowledge. The power and value of oils and their practical use is being rediscovered by women. C'mon, man, do your homework. Put down your child's fidget spinner and redeem the time. Investigate a little, and put forth some effort to make a healthy lifestyle for yourself and your loved ones. Essential oils won't hurt you; they will assist you to heal. They won't make you weak; they actually can help make you strong! Eliminate the excuses now so you won't have regrets later.

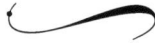

THE LAST DROP

Please, ladies, tread lightly here. You may need to be a bit more tactful when talking to your man about essential oils. I have purposely spoken frankly to the men for you. Your task is to stay patient and gentle. Arguments will not get him to embrace an essential oil lifestyle. Keep the peace.

Guys, no more excuses. It would be healthier to participate in your wife's oil journey. It will be physically, emotionally, and spiritually rewarding. There is significant income potential. Um, really, resisting at this point is a serious waste of time. Don't consider it as "giving in to it" but as "getting in on it!"

"All my life I thought air was free until I bought a bag of chips."

—Anonymous

"We are all born ignorant, but one must work hard to remain stupid."

—Benjamin Franklin

"The more you weigh the harder you are to kidnap. Stay safe. Eat cake."

—Anonymous

"Stubborn is not a word I would use to describe myself; pigheaded is more appropriate.

— *"Michael Bloomberg*

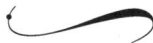

Chapter 9

Your Oil Change Is Due

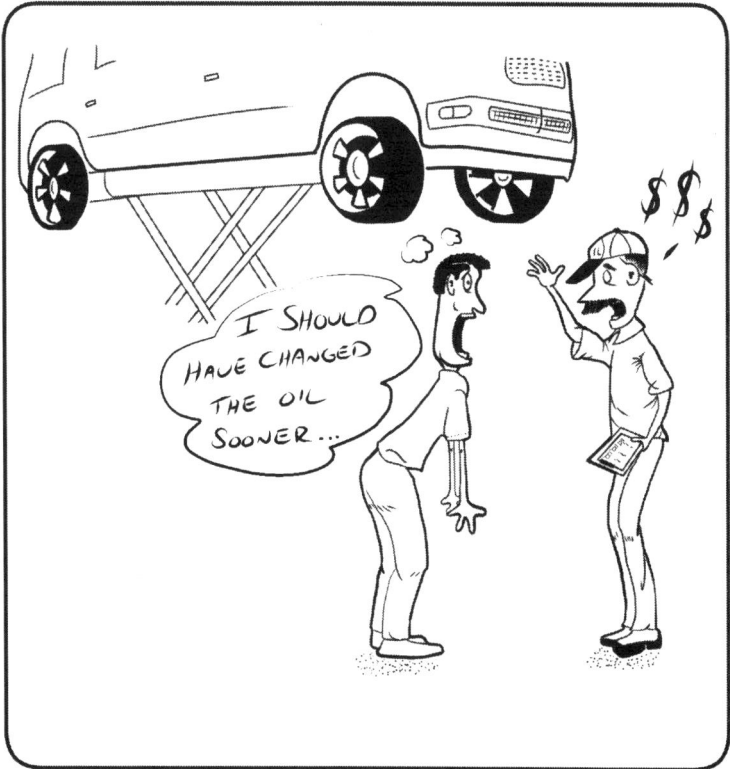

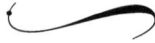

"Create in me a clean heart, O God, And renew a steadfast spirit within me."

—PSALM 51:10

"Worry does not empty tomorrow of its sorrow, it empties today of its strength."

—CORRIE TEN BOOM

"Only those who will risk going too far can possibly find out how far one can go."

—T. S. ELIOT

"To improve is to change; to be perfect is to change often."

—WINSTON CHURCHILL

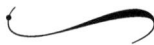

9

YOUR OIL CHANGE IS DUE

W HEN YOUR CAR gets so many miles of wear and tear, there is something very practical and inexpensive that can be done to keep the car from impending engine trouble and is great preventative maintenance. It is simple: change the oil! Changing the oil in your vehicle keeps it running correctly and prevents minor problems from becoming major ones. That "next oil change" sticker with the mileage listed is not on your windshield as a sun shade or to attract insects to the curled-up corners. It is a reminder to change the oil regularly. A little preventative care goes a long way.

And so it is with many a man in regard to his wellness. It's time for an oil change. Like your car, your body feels the effects of a lifetime of wear and tear. Similarly, there are simple maintenance changes you can make that will provide long-term benefits. For some, you are right on time. You have received the oil change reminder and are taking action. For others, this oil change may be severely past due. Like your vehicle, your engine may be burning out. You may feel exhausted, sluggish, or stressed to the max. Don't put off the oil change any longer. Your body and spirit will benefit from the change immensely!

Some men are good with mechanical things and accomplish an oil change themselves. But in this age of video games and people running frenzied from one activity to the other, a great number of men just take it to "the man" to get it done. In either case, the change is getting made, and the average person feels a sense of accomplishment, knowing the completion of this simple maintenance task will add lasting value to the car and fewer complications to their lives. Lasting value and fewer health complications are also true when you make an essential oil change. Many ladies are willing for you guys to do it yourselves and to cheer you on. They will be ecstatic that you are pursuing wellness on your own. Don't get bogged down with whether or not you make changes through your own discoveries or with the assistance of your wife. The key is to make the change. And if you need some extra assistance, there are plenty of wives, mothers, and girlfriends willing to help you with that oil change. Now that's a switch!

With so many facets to consider when changing to essential oil use, you need to put a premium on education. Young Living provides many excellent opportunities to get more education through local, regional, and national events. For men in particular, Founder Gary Young hosted the Iron Will Men's Camp for the past two years. These camps are specifically designed for men to "help you receive the knowledge and tools on how to build confidence, overcome adversity, enhance your life both spiritually and emotionally, and become the man you've longed to be." After a week or two there, you may even be able to leap tall buildings in a single bound!

In addition to classes, camps, seminars, and conventions, there are also several men's Facebook groups to lend support and encouragement. One such group, Essentially Equipped Challenge, contains close to 4,000 men all giving and receiving helpful hints and advice. Be assured that you will not be left alone to drift as you make your oil change.

In this chapter I would like to introduce you to several men who have made an "oil change"—an essential oil change. You can read accounts from average guys who decided that they'd had enough of the old ways, and a change was needed. The following men were reluctant, resistant men who ignored, refused, or just didn't care about essential oils and a wellness lifestyle. They eventually figured out that if they kept going without an oil change, danger was lurking. Everyone can be encouraged through discovering that many men from across the country have similar stories as they moved from skeptics to users. Let me refer to the immortal words of that astute philosopher Rocky Balboa: "If I can change, and you can change...everybody can change!"

This first story comes from my own brother Rob as he related it to me from his corner of the world... Connecticut. Rob's wife, Tammy, had begun to use essential oils, but he remained a dedicated skeptic. She had various stashes of oils around the house, and her knowledge and involvement were growing, but Rob remained resistant. In fact, he sometimes referred to Tammy's oil involvement as a "cult," due in part to her practice of watching videos behind closed doors and at odd hours of the day or night. In spite of many small health gains among family members, Rob held his ground.

YOU CAN LEAD A MAN TO OILS...

His day of enlightenment finally came through the benefits seen in their daughter. It seems their oldest daughter suffered in the spring with terrible allergies, often causing her face to swell and her breathing to labor. She would be confined to indoor activities for a few weeks to avoid the issues. However, this past spring, with the assistance of applications of essential oils, Isabella was able to breathe easily and even play outdoors! Rob admitted this was pretty fantastic. His resistance broke down in the face of this triumph right in his own home. As mentioned in a previous chapter, men respond to the well-being of their children. Now he is actively exploring which oils may help him and encouraging his wife in her essential oil business.

After hearing of my brother's account, I solicited reports from other men who were previously essential oil skeptics. Here are similar stories from other parts of the country containing the same theme:

DAVID HOLDER, FLORIDA

> My wife had been using the oils for months, and I really didn't pay much attention or care one way or the other about them. As I noticed the change in her health and mood, I started

thinking more about them. One day I ran a 12 mile "Tough Mudder" and got the worst blisters I've ever had on the bottoms of both feet. I was in a lot of pain and knew I would be immobile for at least a week. I obviously didn't want that, so we decided to look at a reference guide for some oil protocols to use. I applied oils several times that day and evening before going to bed. When I woke up the next morning, I couldn't believe my eyes! There was no pain or irritation, but most importantly there was a thin layer of skin healed over both blisters! I was flabbergasted and awed by this.

My work is also very stressful, so I often got pretty bad headaches. After using oils for that as well, I rarely get them anymore, and the intensity is far less when I do.

On another occasion I was doing a half marathon with a friend. I was using my oils with the NingXia Red. My friend asked what I was using and could he have some as well. I of course, shared some and off we went. After about 4 miles into the race he stopped and bent over with painful side cramps and had to run to the portable restroom. After a few minutes he came out and said he never had felt so cleaned out in his life! (By the way, we're both in our mid-forties!) I usually have a faster pace but not that day. He was constantly ahead of me and finished minutes before me!

Our lives have been forever changed for the better, and we owe it all to these little bottles of bliss. We will continue to share the ancient powers of the oils that had been long forgotten.

What a clear pattern emerges from David's story: desperation, results, belief, and then sharing with others.

The next story is from my friend Mark. It was his wife, Karen, who first introduced oils to my wife. Mark is a fact-finding, cold, calculating engineer driven by solid data and not given to whim. This is his story as he tells it:

MARK REIGHARD, MISSOURI

I really thought my wife Karen was losing it with all of her hippie voodoo oil stuff. I am an engineer by trade and thought to myself, "this is hokey...if it worked, every doctor out there would be prescribing this rather than the latest pharmaceuticals." But something strange happened. She had really been struggling with her health but all of a sudden she stopped falling asleep in the car, taking afternoon naps and drinking coffee late in the day. She stopped taking her thyroid medicine along with 7 or 8 other pills. She now had more energy all around and was just happier. I didn't believe it, so I asked her to get tested. Everything came back "normal" for the first time in...forever! About that time I had a previously removed growth on my face return, and it was growing quickly. I mentioned going to have it removed again, but Karen said "put some Frankincense on it." "Okay honey" was my response but "good grief" was what I was thinking! I did apply some and three weeks later the growth had shrunk and there was literally no sign of it. Hmm, a couple of pretty good data points.

So after all that I said, "Okay, Coach, I guess I'm willing to try these for real...just tell me what you'd like me to do and I'll do it for three months." So I began routinely applying oils to boost this and support that. I quickly noticed a change in my energy level. She had me drinking more water than usual and we started walking for 20 minutes or so every evening. All of that sort of broke my downward spiral of stress, eating and veg'ing on the couch and got me into a more positive cycle of diet and activity. Long story short, in 3 months I lost 30 pounds and had more energy than I have had in years. I even started running which I had never done in my life!

Ever the engineer, I thought it was likely the placebo effect. After all, I didn't have any real data to prove the effect it had on me. Then along came my annual physical. For the first time in 20 years my cholesterol levels were all within optimal range. My attitude began to change. I began to see the oils as tools that I could use to help fix things. Most men don't like going to the doctor, and I am no exception. So I set out to try and fix something else. For over 20 years I have used prescription sleeping pills (Ambien) to get to sleep every night. "Okay, Coach, what oils will help me sleep?" "Cedarwood and lavender should help," she said. So I give it a try and bam, no more sleeping pills! "Now what about this unsightly mole on my back?" There's an oil for that...bam! What about this headache, muscle ache...BAM!

Now I am a couple of years into this oil journey with Karen. I am still a firm believer in the value of western medicine. However, now I have a healthy appreciation for the benefits of God's natural remedies that have been used for thousands of years. I still seek out and read about clinical trials and studies related to health benefits of essential oils and will always be the one looking for data to support the claims. I have researched and better understand the financial drivers that create tension between natural remedies and the pharmaceutical industry. So now my attitude towards men and oils has completely flipped. These things are tailor made for men. We love tools and we love to fix things. It is typical for us to want to "fix it" when our wives share their issues with us, even when they just want us to listen and have our sympathy. Well, now we have some tools to work with! "Well, Dear, there's an oil for that"...Bam!

Sometimes grasping the significance of oil use is a process rather than a one-time event; however, the pattern of results, belief, and sharing with others remains the same. As a runner, I wish I could cover the 5K distance in one step! Reality says it will take a while and include many steps. I have to keep the end goal in mind and even visualize it as much as I can. But my attention must be to the present steps I am taking as each step is critical to getting me to that end goal. Even when progress is impeded by poor weather or a menacing dog, eventually progress is made. Men making an oil change go through that step-by-step process as well. At times the lack of data, misconceptions, or misunderstandings may impede progress, but again, eventually progress will be made. As they take each step, the final goal comes into focus and confidence grows that it will be achieved.

Did you find that the stories told by these men are similar to your household? I didn't include these stories to be alibis for men to continue putting off the change. These accounts are here to strengthen your resolve to make these changes sooner rather than later and to also see the benefits more quickly. There are many men who have already ended their skepticism.

In fact, some men have been able to incorporate the oils seamlessly into their daily routines. Yes, they have set the bar high for the rest of us (thanks, men), but it proves men can use oils regularly, and it doesn't have to be weird or unmasculine. Their wives are probably beaming with joy each time these men fill a diffuser or rub some oil on their child. Think of how happy your wife will be when you announce you, too, "would like an oil change!"

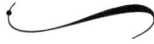

THE LAST DROP

Ladies, I pray these stories give you hope. Many women across the country are facing the same dilemma. Slowly but surely, men are coming around to essential oil use. Take heart that changes are happening in men, and your man may be the next one to take the plunge!

Guys, as you can see, many once-reluctant men are now totally on board with essential oils. Make the change and be refreshed. Imagine the huge burden that will be lifted from your wife. You don't have to wait until you're desperate. Do it now!

"I never make the same mistake twice. I make it five or six times, just to be sure."

—A*NONYMOUS*

"Be decisive. Right or wrong, make a decision. The road of life is paved with flat squirrels who couldn't make a decision."

—A*NONYMOUS*

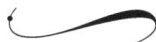

Chapter 10
Taking the Plunge

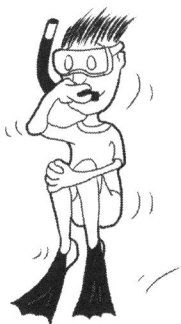

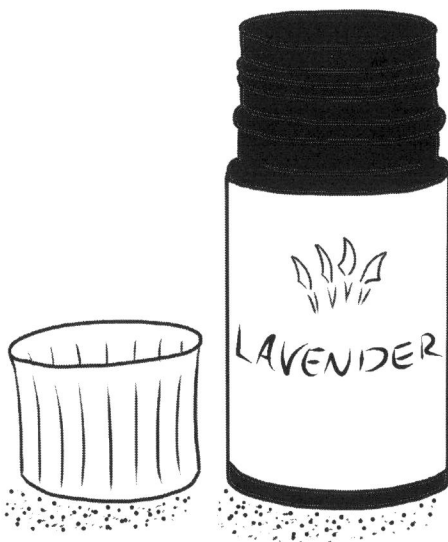

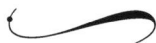

"Give instruction to a wise man, and he will be still wiser, Teach a righteous man, and he will increase his learning."

—*Proverbs 9:9*

"Passion doesn't negate weariness; it just resolves to press beyond it."

—*Priscilla Shirer*

"Don't let your learning lead to knowledge. Let your learning lead to action."

—*Jim Rohn*

"A man of words and not of deeds, is like a garden full of weeds."

—*Benjamin Franklin*

10

TAKING THE PLUNGE

THE GOAL OF this book is to bring sanity to the process of moving a man from oil observer to oil user. When it's all said and done, it is my prayer that your experiences with essential oils will prove to be healthy, encouraging, and family strengthening. Though the approach to this male dilemma has been examined in a sort of tongue-in-cheek fashion, the problem of male reluctance is, to a large degree, real. It is my sincere hope that reviewing it in this manner will take some of the pressure off of the multitudes of women who truly want their men to experience the blessings associated with essential oil use.

The impassioned outcry from many locations about this issue sincerely affected me. As I don't know you all personally, I want to acknowledge the women who spoke to me at the convention and solidified my determination to write this book.

- The woman who spoke to me on the street that first morning was a catalyst.
- The couple from New Jersey whom Diane and I met on the crazy bus ride from the stadium who admitted to the reluctant husband syndrome, and now they are ranked Silver!
- The women in the cosmetic line for three hours with my wife who suggested I call their husbands to get them to come to a convention.
- The woman we met from Oklahoma who so much wanted her husband and son to attend.

All of these and still more who spoke to me about this topic in a class or in the halls represented the sentiments of thousands of women who desperately want their husbands to embrace essential oils and healthier living.

It is my hope that men will also benefit from reading this book by awakening to the wellness they are missing out on and supporting their wives' oily lifestyles. The frustration and hurt women feel when men resist is real. Men, peel back the layers of your wife's emotions and see clearly a woman who loves you and is striving to help you in every way.

In the hope of bringing harmony to your home with regard to essential oils, I offer the following practical suggestions for you. These may help summarize what I've written about and assist you in keeping your efforts in focus.

Tips for women

1. Don't emphasize how wonderful oils smell; emphasize how well they work. Men eventually gravitate toward results.
2. Don't push him to smell or try the oils for no particular reason. Have an outcome in mind.
3. Throwing multiple oils at him for comment or reaction is not recommended. Start with one or two specific oils that will address a simple problem he may be facing, being careful not to overwhelm him with types of oils and information. Slow and steady wins the race.
4. Be clear and concise in the beginning. Too many words without his proper understanding will relegate them to "white noise" status. Brevity will keep his attention.
5. Arguing, guilt trips, and condescending speech will not avail in your effort to get your man to try using essential oils. Let the successful results of the oils in your life and in the lives of myriads of others speak for themselves.

6. Demonstrate to him that your oil use is not a fad by hanging in there for the long haul. Diversify how you use the oils, and let him see their many applications.

7. Before-and-after pictures or experiences will help a man visualize how well the oils work. As seeing is believing, help him to *see* as much as possible.

8. Update him when the oils play a role in supporting your children's health. Men love their children deeply, even if it's unspoken. Positive results in his own children will get his attention and just may win him over.

9. Demonstrate your happiness in the things you are learning and experiencing from your oil use. Don't show him a downcast countenance for his nonuse. Your joy may win him over without a word!

10. Leave a few oil bottles around where he may use them in private. Once you've explained what they are for, he may sneak a drop to test them out.

11. Don't use marital intimacy as a weapon to wound but as a tool to enhance your communication. Arouse his interest in oils, not his resentment to them.

12. Let him know you need his support in gentle ways. Men like it when they are needed, not

cornered. The hero role is something a man can embrace.

13. Encourage men to engage by having couples' classes or even "men only" events. A man will respond if he doesn't feel like a fish out of water. He will put up fewer defenses when he feels safe and in control of the environment. A class full of women may not exactly be his comfort zone.

14. Telling your man how much you love the oils may win him in time. Convincing him that you love him the most may win him sooner!

15. Let this be an area of trust-building in your life. Trust God to bring your man around to essential oils at the proper time and in the best way possible. Trust this man you love to do the right thing.

16. Be grateful. It's contagious.

17. Laugh often. Step back and see the silly excuses of your husband and your bumbling attempts to educate him, and enjoy the ride. You may even want to journal for review purposes later. Hindsight is a source of great humor!

18. Here is a novel idea...talk about his apprehensions! If the opportunity arises, have a conversation about what his specific oil hang-ups are. Don't assume you know. A few minutes spent talking may be enlightening for both of you.

19. Demonstrate interest in the things that he is passionate about. Mutual appreciation will carry a lot of weight.
20. Pray. You have an advantage over him because no matter what he says or how much he resists trying the oils, you can be praying for him. Prayer works in mysterious ways. Trust the Heavenly Father to do the right thing at the right time. He always does!

Tips for men

1. Trust your wife, mother, sister, or girlfriend. These are people in your life who love you and want the best for you. Don't ignore or blow off their advice. They just might know a thing or two that will really help you.
2. Reject the notion that "oils are for women only." This notion is pure nonsense. You will enjoy health benefits, gain wisdom, and be more satisfied.
3. Put a drop of oil on your skin. You will not die.
4. Give the oils a test drive. Target a certain issue and see if the oils can help over time. You may be quite surprised at the results.
5. Keep in mind essential oil use is not hocus-pocus or snake oil magic. Everyone, and every oil, is different. You may get instant results or

you may need time or even a different oil. Be patient.

6. Give your woman some credit for finding something that works. You may not be a big oil user yet, but take satisfaction in knowing her wellness is improving and she desires to help others!

7. Don't treat this oil adventure as a fad but rather as a lifestyle change. Embrace the change in a manner that satisfies your wife and that allows you to enjoy the journey toward wellness.

8. Remember that selling essential oils through network marketing is a legitimate business, not some kind of crazy scheme, pyramid or otherwise! The business is about educating people toward health, not fooling people for wealth.

9. Collect oil data. There are loads of books, blogs, and personal testimonies to build a library of facts to support your oil use and business. Don't force your wife to do all the research for you.

10. Try talking to other men who use essential oils. Find out how they use them. Discover ways they have normalized the use of oils in their daily routine.

11. When you have a health issue, allow your wife to administer some essential oils. You will be glad that she did.

12. Do what you can to support your wife's oil business. Don't crush her with criticism and dash her hopes. Encourage her and serve her, and you'll both be blessed as her business thrives and her soul flourishes. Carry stuff!

13. Revel in the fact that your woman loves you, and her heart is crying out to you to join her in this essential oil venture. Your relationship will strengthen as you move toward wellness together.

14. Step up to the plate! Do the right thing, even if you don't love it. Making tough decisions and taking risks is part of a man's world. Don't abandon that when it comes to using essential oils. You vowed to support your wife—now here's your chance.

15. Belief is a mighty force. Let your wife know you believe in her wellness business dreams. Believe with her, and sometimes for her, when the situation dictates.

16. Celebrate the successes along the way. Everyone needs affirmation. Back up the dump truck and pour out praise and encouragement on your wife. Minimize the discouragements.

17. Keep the healthy things your wife is trying to implement for your good in view and enjoy her passion. It's all *good*!

18. God meant for you to be strong. Adapting, learning, and changing reveals great strength in you. Go for it!
19. Attend a convention with your wife. When you immerse yourself in the essential oil world for a couple of days, you will get your "learn on" and gain a new perspective.
20. This is a great test of your prayer life. Use the opportunity to remove anxiety about essential oils and pray with your wife and for her. Pray for wisdom. Pray for understanding. Pray about your health. Prayer and oils are a powerful combination.

Ladies, won't it be spectacular to see your man using the oils on his own and even requesting that you order more? How fulfilling it will be when essential oils are incorporated in his daily routine. How rewarding it will be as you watch him assemble his own oil stash. Dare to imagine that someday soon, he will be encouraging you to tell others about the oils. He just might even suggest you start or grow your own essential oil business! One day in the near future, you could be booking two tickets to convention instead of one. I envision many women celebrating as men across the country fearlessly tell people about the oils and their many benefits. Picture for a moment men chatting it up with other guys about oils at the workplace or on the golf course. What was once a dream is now within reach. The skeptical male will soon be a thing of the past.

With a little understanding, education, and a whole lot of love, you *can* lead a man to oils!

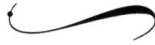

THE LAST DROP

"For all sad words of tongue and pen, the saddest are these, 'It might have been.'"

—JOHN GREENLEAF WHITTIER

"Do you not know that those who run in a race all run, but only one receives the prize? Run in such a way that you may win."

- *I CORINTHIANS 9:24*

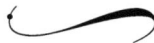

1. Bottle = A miniature glass container of bliss; high multiplication rate; not uncommon to find empties in great quantities.

2. Box = Refers to the only cardboard container that matters in an essential oil home; the carton containing the next order of oils. Upon arrival, causes all household functions to cease.

3. Classes = Stress-inducing gatherings for those preparing; eye-opening venues for newcomers; instructive sessions with the ability to morph into a wide spectrum of activities.

4. Compliant Speech = Rephrasing, avoiding, or skirting truth; manifesting the truth about your health experiences in a veiled way when speaking on the record.

5. Diffuser = A subtle way to get nonusers to use essential oils; a night light; a cause for envy or delight, depending on ownership.

6. Disclaimer = An amusing game played by essential oil speakers or by seminar presenters. Intended to baffle listeners.

7. Downline = The upline for someone else; in need of regular nurturing, encouragement, and inspiration.

8. Drop = A precise measurement of essential oil. Under no circumstance is one to be wasted, or that person faces penalty of death

9. Fragrance = Posh synonym for smell; female lure to essential oils. Can be synonym for "toxic" in less-than-therapeutic-grade oils.

10. NingXia Red = Magical red formula; potentially addicting. Enthusiasts attend swinging club bearing its name that mysteriously appears annually and then vanishes just as mysteriously. What happens at convention stays at convention.

11. Oblivious male = One who lacks mindful attention to the entire essential oil topic. He may in fact be totally unaware. May be found preparing for a Zombie apocalypse.

12. Oil = Refers to pure, potent, therapeutic grade essential oils, not crude oil or motor oil or salad oil; not found in quart containers.

13. Overzealous woman = Fictitious character; no essential oil-using woman would be so impulsive and obnoxious about her passion so as to be given this name.

14. Premium Starter Kit = The irresistible tractor beam that draws people in to an oily lifestyle; Christmas in a box.

15. Reluctant male = One who displays an unwilling-ness, hesitancy, or aversion to getting involved with essential oils. Complains and moans at the first sign of illness; remains helpless until illness passes.

16. Resistant male = One who actively opposes the use of essential oils; may appear angry or sickly, if he appears at all.

17. Skeptical male = One who doubts all things related to essential oil use, including, but not lim-ited to, the need for, regular use of, results, and

incorporation into a toxic free lifestyle. He also believes the world is flat.

18. Team = The group of unorthodox, creative, sensational people you spend time with due to equal essential oil fixation.

19. The Business = Universal transport system that moves people with an entrepreneurial spirit to places of great adventure; needs constant attention.

20. Toxic = Hazardous elements found in places they are not meant to be (i.e., food, household products); those who detract from your goals.

21. Toxin free = Homes and/or products in which all hazardous elements whether chemical or human have been banished.

22. Upline = The downline for someone else; often perceived as role models and mentors; also in need of encouragement.

23. Wellness = Living life with little or no infirmity; slang expression employed by essential oil users to speak compliant lingo.

SEED TO SEAL

it's not a slogan, it's our calling

Young Living knows that producing the highest-quality essential oils starts long before the cap is put on the bottle. That's why our proprietary Seed to Seal® process is the foundation of everything we do. With five careful steps, we make sure only the best products bear the Young Living mark of quality.

SEED: To make the best, we start with the best seeds and botanicals that have been evaluated for their essential oil-producing potential.

CULTIVATE: Our experts travel the world visiting the Young Living farms and our carefully monitored partner growers to make sure cultivation processes meet or exceed the highest standards.

DISTILL: Our gentle, proprietary techniques extract essential oils while preserving their precious constituents.

TEST: To guarantee consistent, verifiable quality, our oils are tested in third-party facilities, as well as in Young Living's own internal labs.

SEAL: Using state-of-the-art equipment, our essential oils are carefully bottled, labeled, and then shipped to members worldwide.

YOUNG LIVING 2016 U.S. INCOME DISCLOSURE STATEMENT

As a direct selling company selling essential oils, supplements, and other lifestyle products, Young Living offers opportunities for our members to build a business or simply receive discounts on our products.

Whatever your interest in the company, we hope to count you among the more than 2 million Young Living members joining us in our mission to bring Young Living essential oils to every home in the world.

What are my earning opportunities?

Members can earn commissions and bonuses as outlined in our Compensation Plan. As members move up in the ranks of Young Living, they become eligible for additional earning opportunities.

This document provides statistical, fiscal data about the average member income and information about achieving various ranks.

RANK	PERCENTAGE OF ALL MEMBERS[1]	MONTHLY INCOME[2]				ANNUALIZED AVERAGE INCOME[3]	MONTHS TO ACHIEVE THIS RANK[4]		
		Lowest	Highest	Median	Average		Low	Average	High
Distributor	94.0%	$0	$941	$0	$1	$12	N/A	N/A	N/A
Star	3.5%	$0	$811	$60	$77	$924	1	15	255
Senior Star	1.3%	$1	$5,157	$197	$240	$2,880	1	22	255
Executive	0.6%	$50	$12,139	$434	$514	$6,168	1	29	253
Silver	0.7%	$262	$25,546	$1,783	$2,227	$26,724	1	36	251
Gold	0.1%	$1,781	$46,800	$4,874	$6,067	$72,804	1	54	240
Platinum	<0.1%	$3,146	$85,993	$12,188	$15,324	$183,888	2	63	238
Diamond	<0.1%	$14,896	$140,333	$22,078	$39,566	$474,792	10	75	251
Crown Diamond	<0.1%	$33,227	$232,581	$44,256	$74,188	$890,256	14	83	236
Royal Crown Diamond	<0.1%	$58,392	$262,864	$155,248	$152,377	$1,828,524	17	106	230

The income statistics in this statement are for incomes earned by all active U.S. members in 2016. An "active" member is a member who made at least one product purchase in products in the previous 12 months. The average annual income for all members in this time was $25, and the median annual income for all members was $0. 51% of all members who enrolled in 2015 did not make a purchase with Young Living in 2016. 57% of all members who enrolled in 2014 did not continue with Young Living in 2016.

Note that the compensation paid to members summarized in this disclosure do not include expenses incurred by a member in the operation or promotion of his or her business, which can vary widely and might include advertising or promotional expenses, product samples, training, rent, travel, telephone and Internet costs, and miscellaneous expenses. The earnings of the members in this chart are not necessarily representative of the income, if any, that a Young Living member can or will earn through the Young Living Compensation Plan. These figures should not be considered as guarantees or projections of your actual earnings or profits. Your success will depend on individual diligence, work, effort, sales skill, and market conditions. Young Living does not guarantee any income or rank success.

[1] Based on a count of all active members in 2016.
[2] Because a distributor's rank may change from month to month, these percentages are not based on individual distributor ranks throughout the entire year, but based on the average distribution of distributor ranks during the entire year.
[3] Because a distributor's rank may change from month to month, these incomes are not based on individual distributor incomes throughout the entire year, but based on earnings of all distributors qualifying for each rank during any month throughout the year.
[4] This is calculated by multiplying the average monthly incomes by 12.
[5] These statistics include all historical ranking data for each rank and thus is not limited to people who achieved these ranks in 2016.
[6] These incomes include income earned from January 1, 2016, and December 31, 2016, but which was paid between February 2016 and January 2017.
[7] Members who do not make at least one product purchase in the previous 12-months have their membership terminated.

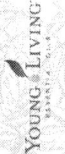

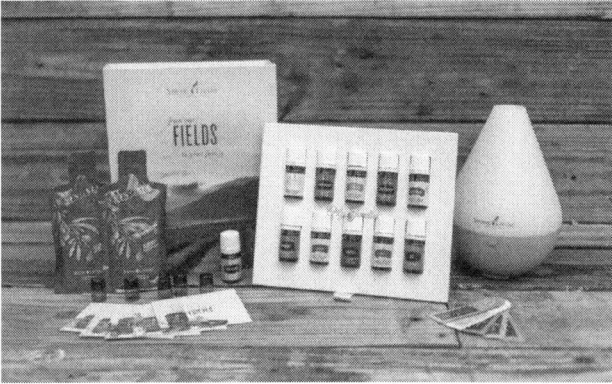

Your Premium Starter Kit Includes:

- Dewdrop™ Diffuser
- Premium Essential Oils Collection:
  - Lavender 5-ml
  - Peppermint Vitality™ 5-ml
  - Lemon Vitality™ 5-ml
  - Copaiba Vitality™ 5-ml
  - Frankincense 5-ml
  - Thieves® Vitality™ 5-ml
  - Purification® 5-ml
  - R. C.™ 5-ml
  - DiGize™ Vitality™ 5-ml
  - PanAway® 5-ml
- Stress Away™ 5-ml
- AromaGlide™ Roller Fitment
- 10 Sample Packets

- 10 Love It? Share It! Sample Business Cards
- 10 Love It? Share It! Sample Oil Bottles
- 2 NingXia Red® 2-oz. samples
- Product Guide and Product Price List
- Essential Oil Magazine
- Essential Edge
- Member Resources
  One or more of the following essential oils may be substituted in the event of sourcing constraints or supply considerations: AromaEase™, Citrus Fresh™ Vitality™, Lemongrass Vitality™, Orange Vitality™, and Tea Tree.

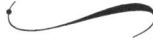

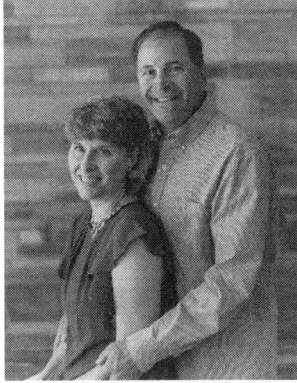

Introducing Ron and Diane Corica

Ron Corica was a skeptical male. He has been happily using essential oils since the fall of 2015. He is a cancer survivor searching for natural remedies. Originally from Connecticut, the family settled in Diane's home state of Missouri, west of St. Louis. Ron has a degree in Christian education from Moody Bible College in Chicago, Illinois. He has been a teacher, counselor, and pastor for over thirty years. Ron has addressed problems men and women encounter through these experiences. Ron is also the owner and manager of his own family business. Very competitive, Ron likes to watch most sports and is an avid runner and fossil hunter. He embraces "the thrill of the hunt!" Ron and Diane love to take road trips together. Diane homeschooled their six children over a twenty-year span. She has been a volunteer horse trainer for fifteen years at Strong Tower Ranch in Missouri. Besides horses Diane loves music, reading, and crocheting; and as a Young Living Executive, she leads the Oil Symphony Team.

- We would LOVE to have you join our Young Living team for education for your health! We offer extensive training tools, effective leadership, and several private Facebook groups for support. If another Young Living member sent you to this book, then check back with them first!

Please feel free to contact me (Diane) with any questions at oilsymphony@hotmail.com, visit my website at www.yldist.com/oilsymphony, or call me at (314) 803-5151.

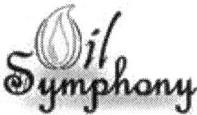

Oil Symphony

Thank you, Friends, for reading this book. I think you'll agree that using essential oils and receiving the health benefits derived from them is fantastic. As much as it is important to inform and enlighten others about essential oils, there is a greater need that affects everyone. The greatest need is not financial security, family harmony, or even physical health. Those are all good things, but each falls short of providing the essential need we all have. That deepest need is to have a relationship with the Creator God, which is only possible through the provision made by the sacrifice of Jesus Christ. All religious activity is man's attempt to do something for God. In reality, God has already done what was necessary to restore relations with every person. All you need to do is believe it. If you would like more information on how you can have that relationship, simply read the blog entitled, *A Greater Love* found on our website: www.yldist.com/oilsymphony. Contact information is also provided there. God bless you!

Made in the USA
Lexington, KY
17 April 2018